Empowered Care

Mind-Body Medicine Methods

Empowered Care

Mind-Body Medicine Methods

Robert Bruce Newman
Ruth L. Miller

A
MEDIGRACE

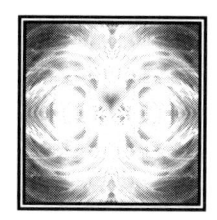

Book

Published by Portal Center Press

Empowered Care: mind-body medicine methods

© 2012 by Robert Bruce Newman and Ruth L. Miller.

Cover Art and Medigrace Books logo by Iona Miller.

A MEDIGRACE BOOK published by
Portal Center Press, Newport, Oregon, 97365

Excerpts from *Transpersonal Medicine* by G. Frank Lawlis, © 1996 by G. Frank Lawlis. Reprinted by arrangement with Shambhala Publications, Inc.

Much of the material in this book may also be found in the book *Calm Healing, Methods for a New Era of Medicine* published by North Atlantic Books, 2006. It is used here with permission of the publisher.

ISBN: 978-1-936902-01-9

Printed in the United States of America.

Mind and body therapies.
2. Alternative medicine.
Mind-Body and Relaxation Techniques.
Mental Healing. WB 880

For all who are ready to experience
a greater kind of health and wellbeing

Contents

Preface vii
PART ONE: THE CONTEXT.. 1
Introduction.. 1
Mind-Body Medicine Comes of Age... 7
    The Unified Mind-Body 8
    Mind-Body Evidence.. 10
    Mind-Body Research and Treatment...................................... 14
Meditation Methods Across Cultures 27
    Shamanic Traditions... 27
    Judeo-Christian Mystic Healing Traditions............................ 29
    Hindu Mystic Healing Traditions 36
    Tibetan Wisdom 39
    Ancient Wisdom, New Possibilities for Healing.................... 44
Mind-based Healing In The United States................................... 45
    Meditation Is Established in American Culture..................... 45
    Mindfulness Meditation.. 46
Meditation Research 51
    Early Research in Other Countries 51
    Meditation Research in the United States.............................. 53
    Psychological Benefits of Meditation..................................... 61
    Physiological Benefits of Meditation 63
    Meditation as a Means for Promoting Wellbeing................... 67
    A New Medical Approach.. 73

PART TWO: A NEW MODEL OF HEALING 75
States of Consciousness—Emerging Understandings 77
    A Continuum 80
    Other Western Models.. 81
    Eastern Models 84
    Meditation Methods & States of Consciousness 88
New Understandings of the Body 93
    The Energetic Mind-Body 94
    The Multiple Bodies of the Human Mind-Body.................... 117
Integrating Models of the Human Mind-Body 127
    Implications Of The Model 131

A New Model of the Healing Process 133
    Illness as a State of Consciousness 134
    Transpersonal Medicine 136
    The Power of Intention 138
    Energy Healing Methods 139
    The Role of Meditation 141
    The Healer 148
    An Integrated Model of the Healing Process 149

PART THREE: METHODS FOR SELF-CARE AND FOR THE
HEALING OF OTHERS 153
Deep Release 155
    The Method 156
    Introduction 157
    The Practice 158
Awareness-Based Energy Breathing 177
    The Method 178
    Introduction 181
    The Practice 182
Guided Imagery 193
    The Method 194
    Introduction 194
    The Practice 195
Releasing the Past; Healing the Present 201
    The Method 201
    Introduction 202
    The Practice 203
Compassionate Breathing (Ton Len) 215
    The Method 217
    Introduction 219
    The Practice 222
Healthcare Methods for the Semi-Comatose and Comatose, and for Near-
Death Care 229
    1. ALZHEIMER'S CARE: TREATMENT FOR THE SEMI-
    COMATOSE 230
    The Method 231
    Introduction 232
    The Practice 232
    2. CARE FOR THE COMATOSE 237
    The Method 237
    Introduction 238
    The Practice 238

3. HEALING IN NEAR-DEATH CARE 243
  The Method 243
  Introduction 244
  The Practice 245

PART FOUR: NEW POSSIBILITIES 249
Transforming Our Paradigm of Illness & Wellness 251
  The Genius & Potential of Self-Care 251
  Opportunities 252
  Transformative Processes 254
Healing the Person, Healing the Planet 257
  The Transpersonal Mind-Body 257
  An Interconnected Whole 259
  Quantum Relationship 260
  Global Consciousness 262
  Prayer, Meditation, and the Maharishi Effect 264
Advancing Medical Options and Medical Science 267

Appendix A The Light Nature of the Energy Body According to Vajrayana Buddhism 271
Appendix B The Issue of Will in Western Culture 275
Appendix C The Material Science of the Light Body 279

Glossary 283
Concise Bibliography of Vajrayana Literature in English 291
End Notes 293
General References 303
Index 308
About the Authors 313
About Medigrace 315

> The species sees itself alive and growing fast
>
> with so much deadly might in its power
>
> it turns faster into the light of its mass.
>
> ~ Robert Bruce Newman

Underlying the physical structure of the universe units of light called photons form and reform into all the potential modes of matter and energy. Experiments have demonstrated that cells regenerate and communicate throughout our biochemical bodies through the exchange of light. Inwardly people seek something called inner light, potentially far more luminous than the radiant activity of atoms. In the revered literature of the spiritual sciences this is called the "clear light"[1] or "ground luminosity."[2] And in the moment before death, when the tendencies of the lifetime have dissolved, the powerful clear light of each life is revealed.[3]

Now, in the early twenty-first century, there is an accelerating realization of the true nature of the human body. It's becoming clear that an experience of inner light may be essential for each person's wellbeing.

As we accept this realization we develop a new model of the healing process—for all forms of care—and we can offer healthcare methods known to empower individuals so they can heal themselves and others.

Preface

To the Reader:

This book expands on and updates one we wrote in 2005, which was published as *Calm Healing, methods for a new era of medicine* in 2006, and is still available through its publisher, North Atlantic Books.

Over the years since the earlier publication we've advanced our work and further defined the healthcare methods being offered. We've created this new book to make some of the more recent work and understandings in the field of mind-body theory and healthcare accessible to more readers.

We've changed the format of that original book, adding and deleting sections, and treating the many references as endnotes, in hopes that the reader will move through the text more easily while still having access to the sources. And, to bring the methods, the model, and the benefits of both into sharper focus, we've.clarified and simplified some of the contextual material.

It's our hope that you will find this new book a helpful and empowering guide to the realm of wellbeing through self-care.

Appreciatively,
Robert Bruce Newman & Ruth L. Miller

PART ONE: THE CONTEXT

The world constantly changes in its inconceivable dimensions and states, and in the late 20th and early 21st centuries change came more rapidly in more areas of life than ever before. In the midst of this rapid and extensive change, many aspects of human life have been transformed, and the field of medicine has experienced a paradigm shift.

In my 30 years of practicing medicine I've found no healing force more impressive or more universally accessible than the power of the individual to care for and cure him- or herself.

~ Herbert Benson[4]

Introduction

Medical science as we know it, called here "scientific medicine," emerged in the late 19th century and flourished during World War II, when the advancement of surgical technology and pharmaceutical interventions led to an innocent confidence that modern scientific medicine could conquer all diseases and solve all health-related problems. This confidence was founded in experience: the remarkable results of high-technology surgery and the widespread effectiveness of antibiotics suggested infinite potential for this new approach.

Scientific medicine is a powerful tool and a generally effective model, through which treatment of acute conditions such as injuries has most often been superb. But there has been a growing dissatisfaction with the prevalent use of drugs and surgery in response to a range of conditions, some of which may have benefited from another approach. Recently, the misuse and overuse of those interventions have become a significant problem, making hospital care one of the leading causes of death, according to the American Medical Association.[5]

There is also growing concern about widespread addiction and reactions to various drugs—both prescribed and illegal. Anxiety and stress have become a pandemic psychophysical condition, engendering excessive dependence on drugs for "killing" pain and coping with unprecedented levels of psycho-emotional illness. As many as 90 percent of all office visits to doctors of conventional medicine during the 1980s and '90s were based on anxiety and stress.[6] Even the medical establishment became concerned about the high incidence of adverse drug reactions, with the American Medical Association reporting that reactions to prescriptions "may be the fourth to sixth leading cause of death."[7]

Through the twentieth century, what is now called allopathic medicine became a technological response to the body and its practitioners were seen by patients and their families as too often lacking compassion. Doctors came to be seen as the victims of a limited and often restrictive medical training preoccupied with applying new drug protocols, largely defined by pharmaceutical corporations. Concern also emerged about the poor health of doctors and nurses, characterized by high rates of drug and alcohol addiction and shorter life spans than normal.

Entering the 1990s, growing dissatisfaction with these potentially dangerous patterns led many Americans to choose practitioners of Complementary and Alternative Medicine (CAM) more frequently than providers of conventional medicine. Their distrust of established models of healthcare and a desire for alternative approaches led to widespread interest in medical arts of other times and cultures, such as acupuncture, homeopathy, and herbal medicine, as well as the science of meditation and emerging mind-body therapies.

The reasons for the transfer of trust are multifold. The CAM providers are typically healthier than establishment medical professionals and they are often more highly trained in the application of their specific modalities, while accepting their limitations. They typically see themselves as healers, rather than authorities, and are very patient-oriented and sensitive to mind-body dynamics. As a result, they more typically express more compassion and healing intention in the care they offer, which are pivotal values for the people seeking alternative healthcare.

In response to this movement, the U.S. National Institutes of Health established a National Center for Complementary and Alternative medicine in 1991, and an increasing number of medical schools have begun to teach CAM modalities. These are signs that a significant shift is occurring in the medical paradigm. In his encyclopedic work, *Planet Medicine*, Richard Grossinger offers a vision of the scope and scale of the changes forthcoming. In the chapter called "The New Paradigm," he says:

> Paradigm shifts are elusive, multidimensional phenomena. In their midst no one can guess how far they will go and what they will eclipse... Holistic health is finally a refraction of environmental awakening, political activism, and a synthesis of Eastern

and Western epistemologies and ethics. It is not first and foremost a medical paradigm... "holistic health" or alternative medicine is merely the faintest glimmering of a new world.[8]

Marilyn Ferguson offered a compelling description of the overall shift our culture is undergoing in her seminal work, *The Aquarian Conspiracy*. In it she described the necessary revolution in the structure of medicine:

> If we respond to the message of pain or disease, the demand for adaptation, we can break through to a new level of wellness... Just as the readiness of a new constituency makes a new politics, the needs of patients can change the practice of medicine... The role of altered awareness in healing may be the single most important discovery in modern medical science.[9]

Larry Dossey, MD, whose books on mind-body medicine have been a major influence in the field, published his model of the "Three Eras of Medicine" in his classic text, *Meaning and Medicine*, in 1993. He defines Era I as scientific medicine, focused on observable "facts" and the diagnosis and elimination of symptoms, through suppression or surgery. Era II medicine, he says, is mind-body medicine, with its focus on methods that can help people take an active role in their health. Era III medicine, said Dossey, is transpersonal medicine, focused on methods that bring people to their innate abilities to heal themselves and others.

As often happens during cultural shifts, all of these "Eras" are in place today. Dossey's Era II and Era III medicine began to emerge simultaneously in America and the West in the 1970s and 1980s and continue to manifest and evolve today. Helping to clarify and define them is the focus of this book.

In their first book, *The Creation of Health*, Caroline Myss and Norman Shealy described the needed revolution in healthcare as a shift of power from the doctor to the patient. Addressing the medicine model that Dossey calls Era I, they say that the doctor is all-powerful, while the patient is passive and completely dependent on the doctor's directives. This, they tell us, is not a psychologically healthy situation for the patient or for the doctor. To shift power from the doctor to the patient, healthcare education and training in mind-body methods would be key.

Another significant model of how the health sciences have had to evolve is offered by Herbert Benson, whose decades of work at Harvard Medical School were pivotal to the emergence of mind-body methods. In his book, *Timeless Healing,* Benson boldly stated that the scientific medical establishment would collapse under the weight of its own problems unless it developed a new model in which self-care was the essential feature. He proposed that if people were educated in the use of mind-body methods, such as meditation, they would be able to take an empowered role in their own health. Consequently, he suggested, pharmaceuticals and surgery would be used only as they supported self-care, which, he declared, needs to be the primary mode of care.[10]

In parallel with these emerging new visions of possibility for medicine, new understandings about the nature of the human body have emerged. Some of these realizations derive from the discoveries of other fields of science, such as quantum physics, cybernetics, electromagnetics, and biophysics. Others explain how it is that the CAM approaches are effective. Still other ideas emerge from western culture's discovery of the wisdom available in the time-tested practices of other cultures.

Marilyn Ferguson was among the first to publish this knowledge in her 1980s journal, *Brain-Mind Bulletin.* Since then, many journals and organizations have continued to explore these alternatives, notably the Institute of Noetic Sciences, the Heartmath Institute, "New Dimensions Radio," Ken Wilber's numerous books, and Michael Murphy's remarkable *Future of the Body* published in 1992.

It is presently 2012. This book presents a set of Era II and Era III methods developed over the past century and drawn from even more ancient traditions. We include methods that have been refined in application to cancer care, cardiovascular care, Alzheimer's care, near-death care, and childbirth—reclaiming great methods from the past and presenting newer ones. The chapters of this book present the background and context for these methods and explore the natural human genius for healing. Our goal is to make people aware of new dimensions of experience by offering new ways to truly heal, to give birth, and to transform death into greater life.

Most of the methods offered here conform to Dossey's Era II model of medicine, but a few epitomize his Era III model. Two of the methods we present are applications of meditation science proven to be of benefit in treating a number of symptoms. One is an application of a proven method of mind-body medicine, refined through many years of use in a variety of applications. Other methods presented here offer a new means of healing that honor the emerging model of the human body.

As of today, more than one hundred training seminars in these methods have been presented in West Coast hospitals, with education credits offered by the California Board of Registered Nursing. In these trainings we've experienced a movement into a new domain of healing, through the power of intention. Participants experience a practical knowledge and sensation of the unified field of which we all are part as they express their intention to affect that field through their new, transformative practice.

The remarkable power of intention has been known for millennia—individually and in groups we are each the nucleus that brings forth the whole—but our culture has tended to ignore it. With the effective action of groups engaged in mind-body healing, an exponentially increasing force for healing has begun to emerge.

Our culture has meanwhile achieved instantaneous worldwide communication via satellite, the computer, and telephone. The integration of these two factors brings us into a personal/global state that holds the potential for worldwide mind-body healing. As a result, the new form of medicine we are describing here has the potential for individual and mass healing that can carry the individual practitioner into an unprecedented domain of wellbeing.

Mind-Body Medicine Comes of Age

For thousands of years and across human cultures, there has been an understanding that awareness—which has been called mind, consciousness, soul, spirit, essence, and many other names— is fundamental to all human existence, and that the human mind has an effect on both body and environment.

In the ancient Vedic traditions, the universe is described as intelligent energy, which, in Sanskrit, is called Brahman, which has been condensed and organized into matter through the activity of consciousness. The several thousand-year-old text called *Mundaka Upanishad* states:

> By energism of Consciousness Brahman is massed; from that Matter is born and from Matter, Life and Mind and the worlds.

This understanding is the basis for the Hindu and Buddhist principle that matter, and all the life forms that have evolved within it, is *maya*, which means changeable, malleable. Our experience only seems real, but is a projection—because, ultimately, awareness, or Brahman, is the only reality, being timeless. Matter is a temporary, changing, form, occurring only in the presence of mind.

Plato's realm of the Ideal, out of which imperfect forms may be perceived, is consistent with this model. His model suggests that all we perccive is an imperfect formulation of the Ideal, which is eternally in potential. Much of early Christian (and modern New Thought) philosophy is based on this model of reality.

And from Siberia to Mexico to Australia, shamans' journeys lead to the same conclusion: beyond the "worlds" of matter and illusion lies a reality beyond our perception, containing the potential of all possible forms of material existence. Anthropologist Carlos Castaneda tells us that the Yaqui shaman Don Juan Matus, following ancient Toltec traditions, called that reality the *nagual*, and consistently warned Carlos to be careful lest his own mind, unintended, create undesirable forms within it.

According to these ancient traditions from around the world, then, the activity of mind has power. It manifests form out of the substance of the universe, both in the body and outside it.

That Western science has not explored these matters until recently is the result of a historical process that began with the work of René DesCartes in the 17th century. Because of him, study of the physical world was given to "natural philosophers" and scientists, while, after centuries of control over all realms of knowledge throughout Europe, study of the realm of spirit was retained by the Church and theologians. It's only been in the past few decades, since the power of the religious institutions has diminished, since the secularization of national and community life across Europe and the Americas, that scientists have dared to outwardly explore the realms of consciousness, or spirit. And it wasn't until the twentieth century, when, unexpectedly, the new sciences of quantum physics and cybernetics made it essential to explore these areas, that the old injunction finally fell away.

The Unified Mind-Body

Today, the evidence is clear. In the very "hard" science of physics, it's been proved over and over again that all matter and energy is changeable, and that the mind of the observer affects results. And in the life sciences, the role of mental activity in physiological function is no longer denied.

As a result, a new vision of the mind-body begins to emerge in the medical model. The science of psychoneuroimmunology epitomizes that vision as it combines the fields of anatomy, physiology, chemistry, psychology, and biophysics. It emerged largely out of research into the cause and cure of AIDS, and it has been applied in more and more situations since. In these applications, the evidence demonstrates that the state of mind and emotions of the patient affect the activities of individual cells and the overall state of the body.

Perhaps the best known articulator of this new understanding is Dr. Deepak Chopra, a Western-trained physician and former chief of staff of the New England Memorial Hospital, who came to understand, through the evidence presented to him in his practice, that there was far more to the healing process than his scientific background could explain. His first exploration of the potential for unifying mind and body, entitled *Quantum Healing*, has become a classic. In it he traces his journey from a purely Western view of the body and mind as separate and unrelated, through quantum physics, and into the ancient traditions of the land of his birth.

He describes his first inexplicable experience as occurring when he was an intern with an aged, dying man who had only days or hours to live, but who, when the youthful doctor Chopra blithely told him he'd see him when he returned from another assignment, held on to life for several weeks until his favorite doctor came and saw him again—and died almost immediately thereafter. Chopra also tells the reverse kind of story in the book, for example, the man who had lived comfortably with a tumor in his lungs for six years—until he was told it was cancer, at which point he became very upset and died shortly thereafter.

Chopra explains these stories with the comment that our cells "are always willing to cooperate with the mind's instructions." He tells us, "The whole body is a 'thinking body,' the creation and expression of intelligence."[11]

In a later book, entitled *Creating Health*, Chopra states:

> The real you is the arrangement, the organizing power, the knowledge, the intelligence, the impulse of consciousness that designs material stuff to give the appearance of you. That is the only reality worthy to rank as you in your completeness. It is nonmaterial, whole, dynamic, and yet utterly stable, and infinite in its capacity to evolve.[12]

Chopra's exploration of this model of human beings has led him far from traditional medicine, into the investigation of complementary and alternative treatments now gaining respect in the U.S.[13]

Another major contributor to the cultural acceptance of a unified body and mind has been Candace Pert, the microbiologist with the National Institutes of Health who was able to identify and establish the role of neuropeptides in communicating between cells in the body. According to Pert, these "molecules of emotion" appear everywhere in the body, in trillions of cells, almost simultaneously with whatever stimulus is affecting the emotions. Each emotion has a different set of neuropeptides associated with it, and each set of neuropeptides provides a particular set of instructions to the cells. Even a memory of an event can call forth these chemicals into every part of the body, causing all of our cells to react as if the event were occurring here and now. Her book, *Molecules of Emotion*, firmly established the scientific basis for the effects of thoughts and feelings on the activity of individual cells, throughout the body. and her contribution to the film *What the BLEEP Do We Know!?* has made these ideas accessible to the general public.

On the basis of her research, she concluded that "the subconscious is the body,"[14] suggesting that all of our memories and deeply held assumptions and beliefs are embedded in the cells and intercellular systems of the body.

Molecular biologist Bruce Lipton, seeking to discover the "brain" of the cell, has discovered that, in fact, it is not the nucleus of the cell (which he calls "the gonads," responsible only for reproduction), but the complex outer membrane that governs the cell's activity. In the process, he has been able to describe precisely how the neuropeptides affect the workings of individual cells. In a series of lectures over the past two decades, and in his book, *Biology of Belief*, Lipton graphically demonstrates how both the chemical and the electromagnetic signature of chemicals "unlock" the receptors on the cell membrane. These, in turn, control the chemicals and activities of organelles within the cell. As a result, he says, the energy of a thought, as well as the chemical structures precipitated by our thoughts and feelings, can change the functioning of a cell.[15]

The implications of this model for medicine are staggering. With thoughts changing cellular function, we need no longer look for a physical cause for any particular set of symptoms, but rather to an underlying mental imbalance or emotional disturbance. Further, the presence of physical distress, such as infection or muscle strain, is no longer the focus of our medical intervention, but the indicator of whether or not balance has been restored.

Mind-Body Evidence

In *The Future of the Body*, an exhaustive compilation of the published research on human development, healing, and consciousness, Michael Murphy points out that "psychophysical changes" are far more common than we normally assume, noting that bodies often "rely on common modalities of change," in "largely dissociated processes." He suggests that "Hysterical stigmata and false pregnancy demonstrate the... precision with which highly charged images can shape somatic processes."[16]

The Placebo Effect

Murphy goes on to state:

> Placebo effects and spiritual healing, too, depend on suggestive imagery, as well as expectation of success, the deliberate or covert practice of healing affirmations, health-mimicking behaviors, and confidence in… processes.[17]

In his groundbreaking book, *Anatomy of an Illness*, Norman Cousins, the popular former editor of The Saturday Review, set forth a theory of medicine that earned him a place on the University of California at Los Angeles Medical School faculty. Cousins had experienced a serious illness that he was able to overcome through a series of actions that made sense to him but were not recognized as having any significant medical value in themselves. When, upon recovery, he described his self-treatment in an article, more than one noted physician jeeringly ascribed his newfound health to "the placebo effect."[18]

It's interesting to consider this statement in light of the fact that, in tests of a new medication, the goal is always to find out how many more people find relief from their symptoms from the medication than from the "placebo" ("placebo" means "sweet word" or "I will please" and is usually offered in the form of a "sugar pill" or equally ineffective treatment).

In most studies, the "expected" rate of relief from the placebo is 30+ percent: that is, about a third of the people in such tests recover, or have a significant reduction in symptoms, simply by taking the placebo. This is even more interesting when one understands the rules of such tests: the new medication must show results that are "significantly higher" than the placebo—where a "significant difference" is typically defined as 1%, 5%, or 10%. This means that a "clinically tested" medication is one that has been demonstrated to show results only slightly higher than the placebo!

Cousins was intrigued by the possibilities and did some research of his own. As documented in his book, he came to the conclusion that "the history of medicine is actually the history of the placebo effect."[19] Reviewing the "grim array of potions and procedures" medical practitioners have applied to illnesses over the centuries, ranging from using leeches for "bleeding" a patient to placing hot stones or irons on the body, from force-feeding concoctions of herbs and roots to bombarding the body with radiation, he began to see that

> ...people were able to overcome these noxious prescriptions, along with the assorted malaises for which they had been prescribed, because their doctors had given them something far more valuable than the drugs: a robust belief that what they were getting was good for them. They had reached out to their doctors for help; they believed they were going to be helped—and they were.[20]

This research continues to be supported by several texts on the subject since, the results of which pepper the internet.

In fact, in a recently released, highly publicized book called *The Emperor's New Drugs*, Harvard psychologist Irving Kirsch points out that there is so little difference between the results of anti-depressant drugs and the placebos that most such drugs may in fact be working as placebos.[21] This book has led to an amazing number of internet blogs, posts and tweets, as people come to realize that it may not be the drug they're taking, but the fact that they're taking one, that's making the difference.

The Power of Belief

Today, as always, it doesn't take long for healing practitioners to discover that it's not possible to talk about any particular human body without talking about the mind associated with that body.

Our thoughts and feelings, our attitudes, and our expectations have all been demonstrated to affect the state of our immune system, our rate of healing, our responses to medications and procedures, and the various cycles and interactions going on within our bodies from moment to moment. So, although the term "psychosomatic" ("psycho" referring to mind and emotions and "somatic" referring to the physiology and anatomy of the body) is often used to discount a set of symptoms as "all in one's head," many medical practitioners—most visibly represented by Deepak Chopra, Larry Dossey, Andrew Weil, and Norman Shealy—have come to accept that virtually every symptom is psychosomatic: a function of the interaction of both mind and body.

This understanding is the basis for the set of methods called "mental healing" that were established in the U.S. by Phineas

Parkhurst Quimby in the 1850s. Having overcome a terminal illness through means that had nothing to do with medicine, Quimby, like Cousins, began to experiment and investigate. His process led him into the realm of hypnosis (then called "mesmerism"), which helped him see the power of the mind's action on one's own body and on the bodies of others. Giving up hypnosis as a practice, but aware of the effect of a powerful mind on a receptive one, Quimby began to speak out against doctors and preachers who told people they were sick or undeserving, saying they were causing the very illnesses they were attempting to prevent. His approach, helping patients see the underlying mental cause for their physical symptoms and then changing the mental process, was so successful that a whole mental healing movement (including Louise Hay's much later work) was built on it.

In the late 20th century a Canadian physician, Gabor Maté, applied Bruce Lipton's understanding of how the cell works with belief in his work with addictions and attention deficit disorders (ADD). In the process Maté came to understand that stress, and the beliefs underlying the stressors, is directly related to these and other forms of illness. In *When The Body Says No,* his powerful exploration of the subject, he says, "A major contributor to the genesis of many diseases… is an overload of stress induced by unconscious beliefs."[22]

>These are unconscious beliefs, embedded at the cellular level. They "control" our behaviors no matter what we may think on the conscious level. They keep [our bodies] in shut down, defensive modes or allow us to open to growth and to health.[23]

He lists the most damaging beliefs as:
1. I have to be strong.
2. It's not right for me to be angry.
3. If I'm angry I will not be lovable
4. I'm responsible for the whole world.
5. I can handle anything.
6. I'm not wanted—I'm not lovable.
7. I don't exist unless I do something; I must justify my existence.
8. I have to be very ill to be taken care of.[24]

Experiences that challenge these, he says, take on the physiological equivalents of survival issues, and the body reacts as if there's a life or death situation at hand, shutting down many health supporting systems to deal with them.

Mind-Body Research and Treatment

Once the split between mind and body has been bridged, many lines of inquiry are open—even outside the health sciences. From anthropologists like Gregory Bateson (*Steps to an Ecology of Mind* and *Mind and Nature*) to physicists like Fritjof Capra (*The Tao of Physics* and *The Web of Life*), Brian Swimme (*The Universe Is a Green Dragon*), Amit Goswami (*The Self-Aware Universe* and *The Physics of the Soul*) and Bob Toben and Fred Alan Wolfe (*Space-Time and Beyond*), popular scientific literature has proliferated with experiments, explanations, and theories seeking to unify our experiences of body and mind.

Energy-Based Models

A fascinating line of experimentation began in the late 1950s, when Bernard Grad and his colleagues at McGill University in Canada did a series of tests of the effects of "laying on of hands." In these tests, a self-described "healer" held containers in which mice who were surgically wounded had been placed. The results showed that those mice healed significantly faster and with fewer complications than did the control group. When the same person held containers of water that would be used on barley sprouts, the plants grew taller and stronger than those in control groups. In later experiments, the researchers had other people hold the water containers and found that the plants whose water had been held by people diagnosed with significant psychological problems actually did more poorly than those whose water containers had been held by "healthy" people.

These tests and others described by Grad in the *International Journal of Parapsychology* were not well known, but Peter Tompkins and Christopher Bird's book describing similar tests, called *The Secret Life of Plants*, became a bestseller in the 1970s.

During that same decade, Dolores Krieger, professor of nursing at New York University, began to teach and encourage scientific studies of a technique she called Therapeutic Touch (also known as "TT"), which is based on a similar idea. A trained practitioner learns to place a hand on or slightly above a wound or damaged area of the body, learning to "feel" the problem there and "send" healing "energy" to the area.

Tens of thousands of people around the world have been taught the technique, many of whom are registered nurses, rigorously trained in the rules and principles of traditional chemical and mechanical Era I medicine. The popularity of TT among nurses is evidence of their belief in the inherent capability to heal and their desire to help people directly, beyond the limits of Era I medical protocol. In clinical trials and many documented cases, TT has been established as a significantly effective tool. As one nurse describes her experience:

> I started practicing TT 15 years ago and used it for a few years before I began to sense energetically. Even now, I don't... sense many of the things my beginning students do. So why did I keep on practicing? Because I could see that people I worked with were experiencing the relaxation response, pain relief, accelerated wound healing, mental clarity, emotional balance, and/or spiritual connection.[25]

About the same time that Dr. Krieger was introducing Therapeutic Touch to nurses, another hands-on healing method, called Reiki (which means "universal life energy" in Japanese) was being introduced from Japan by way of Hawaii. The method involves setting an intention to have energy flow through the body and into the patient to restore balance and harmony in the mind-body. Again, thousands of people have been trained in the technique, many of them licensed massage therapists and an increasing number of nurses and surgeons. As with TT, Reiki practitioners are trained to place a hand on, or slightly above, the body, sense the need, and send healing "energy" into damaged areas. Most have experienced the kind of results described by the nurse, above.

Several randomized, double-blind studies of such "hands-on" healing techniques have been completed, with large numbers of subjects. In the best-known such study, conducted by D. Wirth in 1990, non-contact TT (that is, when the practitioner holds the hands above the body, at the edge of a perceived "field," without actually touching the skin) significantly accelerated the rate of healing for deep skin wounds.[26] These and a number of other studies are reviewed by R. D. Hodges on the website, www.thehealingtrust.org-uk, with a summary stating that, even taking into account often poorly designed experiments, the evidence was irrefutable that healings based on intentional directing of energy are real.

Interest in an energy-based healing method from China called *Chi Gung, Ki Gung,* or, sometimes, *Qi Gong* (all pronounced "chee kung") has been growing exponentially, as well. In this method, which is closely related to the more familiar *Tai Chi Chuan,* one moves one's body in ways that facilitate energy movement while visualizing the energy entering, moving through, and supporting organs or tissues that are weak or diseased. The movement provides a kinesthetic, as well as visual, focus for imagery—and also a means for immediate feedback from the body as energy flows are visualized and felt. This integration of several modalities in one method has proved powerful for many of its practitioners—both for healing and for maintaining a sense of wellbeing.

Remarkable results from the use of this method have been documented by many researchers and brought to public awareness by Gregg Braden in his popular book and video, *The Isaiah Effect.* Among the more recent results from the use of *Qi Gong* that are reported in journals, books, and on the web include:

- increased blood circulation, balance, and flexibility, derived from the movements involved in the practice, as well as
- decreased rate of stroke and increased rate of improvement from various surgeries, and
- heightened responsiveness to anaesthesia across large groups of practitioners over several decades.[27]

Less well supported by the research, though anecdotal evidence is available from many sources, are assertions that masters of the practice are able to reduce the size of tumors in others and also to increase the electromagnetic fields generated by living tissue without touching the patient or the material.[28]

Many organizations and websites have been established over the past decades to further awareness of the effectiveness of such methods. One of them, The Healing Trust, in England, maintains the

Mind-Body Medicine Comes of Age

website www.thehealingtrust.org-uk. On it, they proclaim that all holistic healing is, in fact, spiritual healing in the most general sense:

> The word Spiritual originates from the Latin 'spiritus' meaning 'breath of life'.
>
> Healing can be defined as regaining balance of mind, body and/or emotions.
>
> Spiritual Healing is a natural energy therapy that complements conventional medicine by treating the whole person—mind, body and spirit. Healers are thought to act as a conduit for healing energy, the benefits of which can be felt on many levels, including the physical.[29]

In the 21st century, considerable work has been done to establish the existence of an energy field around and within the mind-body system—an energy field that is affected by and affects other energy fields, both human and nonhuman. The film *The Living Matrix* provides beautiful illustrations of how this works and documents a number of experiments on the effects. In it, we see people's physiology changing a few seconds before they see a randomly selected picture of an emotionally charged image, in a series of experiments done at the Institute of Noetic Sciences (IONS)—suggesting that, somehow, the mind-body perceives and reacts to information before the physical perceptual system takes it in.

The film also shows IONS experiments in which positive feelings and thoughts focused on a person are correlated with positive changes in that person's physiology—even when the two people cannot see or hear each other. In addition, work at the Institute of Heartmath is documented in which the pattern of vibration in the energy field around and within the body is shown to be governed by the vibration pattern of the heart, which in turn is shown to vary in the presence of loving intention.

Biofeedback: Demonstration of the Unified Mind-Body

During the late 1960s and early '70s, the idea that the cybernetic learning process of "instant feedback" could be used to assist people dealing with health issues emerged in the popular mind. The Biofeedback Research Society was founded in 1970, and by the mid-1980s thousands of articles on the subject had been published.

Working with the Menninger Foundation in Kansas during the 1970s, Elmer and Alyce Green began to apply these ideas to some common, but difficult-to-treat, health conditions. They set up a series of experiments that let patients observe changes in various recording devices to which they were "hooked up." Many people, children especially, loved the experience of changing the graph on a screen or sheet of paper, generating a tone, or moving a needle on a meter, simply by changing the way they thought or felt. With EEGs, blood-oxygen meters, bloodpressure monitors, stethoscopes, and galvanic skin response (electrodermal activity) meters, the Greens and others taught hundreds of people to adjust their heart rate and rhythm, their circulation, their blood pressure, and even their brain-wave patterns.

It rapidly became clear that, given immediate information about the results of their effort, people could learn to control many normally "involuntary" processes in the body. As they continued their research with other types of scanners and monitors, the Greens concluded, "it may be possible to bring under some degree of voluntary control any physiological process that can continuously be... displayed."[30]

In the many tests and experiments that followed, and in practical application, such "biofeedback" (BF) techniques have been used effectively with a wide variety of health conditions. The InteliHealth website (www.InteliHealth.com) lists the following conditions as amenable to BF therapy:

- tension headaches and migraine
- circulatory limitations, such as Raynaud's disease
- digestive disorders, including constipation
- incontinence, both urinary and fecal
- hypertension (high blood pressure)
- cardiac arrhythmias (abnormal heart rhythms)
- addictions
- epilepsy
- sleep disorders
- PMS (premenstrual syndrome)
- ADD, ADHD (attention deficit disorders)

Mind-Body Medicine Comes of Age

• panic and anxiety disorders

The InteliHealth site also lists several other, more severe conditions related to spinal cord injuries, paralysis, and others, stating that each year, new illnesses are added to the list of health problems that may respond to biofeedback therapy.

The Mayo Clinic website (www.MayoClinic.com) adds to this list the following:

• asthma

• hot flashes

• nausea and vomiting associated with chemotherapy

The Mayo Clinic site further states that biofeedback therapy "can reduce, or even eliminate, your need for medication... help conditions that have not responded to medication... helps put you in charge of your own healing..."

In their exhaustive bibliography of Complementary and Alternative Medicine (CAM) Barrows and Jacobs state:

> Children seem to have a particular aptitude and enthusiasm for this therapy. The resemblance that BF shares with video and computer games has been used to great advantage. Also children have less skepticism about this therapy and learn more quickly than most adults.[31]

In *The Future of the Body* Murphy points out that the essential principles of biofeedback are not new. Children have always used various kinds of toys and play to learn motor skills. Anecdotal accounts of individuals controlling their heart rates and muscle responses have been the topic of stories and articles throughout human history. Speech therapists have used various forms of immediate feedback to train those who are hearing- and speech-impaired for nearly a century. The Mowrers introduced an alarm system triggered by urine to end bedwetting in the 1930s. Others during the same period demonstrated the capacity to learn to totally relax a single muscle.[32]

Still, the dominant paradigm of science and medicine has been that there is little, if any, connection between the autonomic nervous system and conscious thought—and few physicians are taught the principles of biofeedback in their medical training.

One interesting application of BF techniques has been in the modification of brainwave patterns. Increased alpha-wave activity, associated with increased overall wellbeing, has sparked public interest, especially when EEG patterns of experienced Zen meditators were shown to have elevated alpha-wave patterns and the public assumed that the "alpha state" and mystical experience were synonymous.

However, Murphy's assessment of the research is that there is little connection between the level of alpha-wave activity and the experience of mystical states.[33] This relationship is made clear as increases in theta, beta, and asymmetrical patterns of multiple wave levels across the hemispheres are achieved using BF techniques.

Murphy and the Greens are adamant that the primary utility of biofeedback is self-awareness and self-regulation through volition, resulting in a reduced need for medication. And the effectiveness of a BF-based computer video game developed in the mid 2000s called "Journey to Wild Divine" as part of a treatment program for hypertension and other blood pressure related disorders confirms their assertion. It provides an easy and entertaining way to discover how to manage pulse, heart rate, blood pressure and galvanic skin response.

The Effects of Imagery

Visualization and guided imagery emerged as a tool with wide-ranging uses in the 1970s, when a powerfully effective book by Robert Masters and Jean Houston, called *Mind Games*, provided a series of guided group processes for moving from minimal capacity to visualize to instantaneous achievement of deep-trance states and journeys. Shakti Gawain's guide, *Creative Visualization*, was a very popular text through the 1980s, frequently on required reading lists in colleges and universities—even in usually conservative business schools.

By the mid-'80s, both the research and the popular literature were announcing that the process of imagining something fully could have as profound an effect on the mind-body as doing the same activity physically.

The use of visualization as a tool for controlling or eliminating symptoms of disease came into popular awareness in the late 1970s, with the work of Carl Simonton and his cancer support groups. He reported numerous cases in which children and adults were able to reverse tumor growth, relieve pain and pressure, and restore the use of limbs by visualizing processes in the body.

Simonton's conclustion was that imagery therapy can be an effective medical factor, recognizing that the patient's healing intention is essential to its success. It communicates with the mind-body from the inside to help heal.[34]

The power of the imagery used depends on the patient and on transpersonal factors beyond ordinary consciousness. Simonton encouraged the use of meaningful symbols as much as possible. For many of his patients, therefore, white blood cells became soldiers, fighting off the alien hordes, or they were tiny bulldozers carving out the mountain of the tumor and hauling away their loads. For others, the bone marrow became factories, producing healthy blood cells of all types, or the blood vessels became rivers, flowing toxins out to the "port" of the kidneys and bladder.

In this process, one relaxes the body to elevate the alpha-wave activity of the brain and allow an internal experience of visual, auditory, and other sense-related images—drawn initially from memory and imagination. As Jeanne Achterberg put it:

> ...messages have to undergo translation by the right hemisphere into nonverbal or imagerial terminology before they can be understood by the involuntary or autonomic nervous system... imagery... is the medium of communicating between consciousness and the internal environment of our bodies...[35]

The visual symbols used are rendered more effective by the emotional "load" they carry.

Frank Lawlis, a psychiatrist using imagery and other approaches in his pain clinic, found visualization processes particularly helpful in working with his patients. He found support for his experience in the research literature:

> ...the research evidence continues to grow, showing that a patient's imaging can have a positive influence on the healing process in such conditions as birth pain, diabetes, breast cancer, arthritis, migraine and tension headaches, pruritic eczema, acne vulgaris and treatment of severe burns.[36]

Part of Lawlis' success lay in the fact that he didn't insist on "visualization" but, rather, worked with the whole range of senses, building on the faculty of eidetic imagery. Visual imagination has great potential, but so does auditory imagination. Some people feel limited with visual imagination but may make important use of audio-guidance. Imagery therapy is therefore enhanced by the use of methods that access inner senses of people who have limitations in visual-imaginal or auditory-imaginal therapies. In this way, imagery medicine can provide new ways to work with imagination and mind in mind-body medicine.

This expansion from the strictly visual to the other senses has the effect, as Masters and Houston point out in *Mind Games*, of engaging the full mind-body system in the process:

> The most powerful imagery for people suffering from chronic pain is kinesthetic in nature... dependent on proprioceptive faculties of our mind-body... the pleasure we derive from dancing or playing a sport... asking patients to feel their heart relaxing, slowing down, radiating warmth out to their hands and feet as they picture themselves moving slowly around a warm, crackling campfire on a summer beach...and the blood pressure normalizes.[37]

The more senses that are engaged, the more effective the process is in persuading the mind-body that the experience is "real." Vividly imagined experiences, including odors, sensations, felt movements, sounds, and tastes, as well as colors, depth, and emotional responses, are, according to Masters and Houston and other researchers, the most effective, by far.

The Methods section in Part Three of this book provides more specific guidelines for using imagery,

Transpersonal Approaches

The field of transpersonal studies emerged in this country as a result of the human potential movement of the 1960s. Formally, the Association for Transpersonal Psychology (ATP) split off from the Association for Humanistic Psychology in the early 1970s, as an increasing number of scholars from many disciplines began to explore and explain various cultural phenomena, personal experiences, and spiritual traditions that seemed to transcend the mind-body model of the human being that was dominant in that period.

As Lawlis describes it, transpersonal psychology:

> ...depicts evolutionary growth as coming from beyond the self, as a power larger or bigger than the individual . . . The basic tenet of this approach is that the destiny of humanity is the evolution of the human spirit . . .
>
> Transpersonal psychology is both a practice and a field of research. As a practice, transpersonal therapists ...assume within each individual planes of wisdom beyond the primary intellectual strength of the ego. They use therapeutic strategies that attempt to bring out from inner sources the knowledge of the unconscious... [The transpersonal therapist] views healing as the result of harmonizing and balancing the mind-body-spirit dynamics within a person's sphere of being... It sees fellowship with others—community—as one of the strongest influences on our own transformational potential.[38]

Among the disciplines contributing to this relatively new field of study are anthropology, psychology, communications studies and cybernetics, religious studies, and consciousness research. The major focus of the research has been understanding the ways that human experience is affected by external influences that have not been measurable by physical means. Thus, distance healing, meditation, shamanic practices, and the "group consciousness" of organizations and communities have been typical topics at conferences and in journals. Roger Walsh, Frances Vaughan, Joanna Macy, and Angeles Arrien are among the best-known researchers in this field, known through their books describing the models and processes of many cultures and therapies that contribute to the field.

The shamanic traditions of indigenous cultures around the world are a significant part of the Transpersonal focus. Shamanic practices have been increasingly recognized as offering us far more than "witch doctors" and "placebos" as they rely heavily on the unification of mind and body in the healing process. Across various cultures and training methods, they typically include:

- rituals to relieve anxiety and stress, encouraging the patient to relax and release normal patterns of thought.

- laying on of hands,
- herbs and crystals, and
- rhythmic music and movement to bring the mind and body into harmony with the vibrations associated with healing.
- visualization as a means for gaining insight into, and power over, the condition being experienced.

We'll talk more about these traditions in the next chapter.

Noetics

During the same years that ATP was coming into existence, astronaut Edgar Mitchell returned from his journeys in space determined to understand more fully the nature of consciousness. With the support of friends and colleagues, he launched the Institute of Noetic Sciences (IONS). The mission of IONS is to facilitate and communicate scientific research regarding the previously discounted and misunderstood experiences called, variously, "mystical," "psychic," and "spiritual."

In 1976, Willis Harman was appointed director of IONS. A retired engineering professor who had become concerned about the long term effects of technology, he had created the futures studies groups at Stanford Research Institute (now SRI International). There he led a number of research projects that included people like Joseph Campbell and Margaret Mead to determine the role that consciousness plays in culture change. Under his leadership both SRI and IONS were established as major contributors to understanding such phenomena in the scientific and lay communities.

Over the years IONS has engaged in a number of intriguing research projects, including, among many others:

- A study on distant healing intention to help late-stage AIDS patients, published in the *Western Journal of Medicine*;
- A study on the possible effects of Qi Gong on brain-tumor cells in a state-of-the-art laboratory setting that continues under the sponsorship of the National Institutes of Health;
- A study comparing a distant healing vs. control group (no distant healing) with a placebo group on acceleration of wound

healing in women with breast cancer by Marilyn Schlitz, PhD, Harriett Hopf, MD, and Cassandra Vieten, PhD;

- A study of the physiological synchronization between healer and patient involved the development and use of neurophysiological techniques to evaluate hypotheses emerging from the field of mind-body medicine by Leanna Standish, PhD, Deepak Chopra, MD, and Marilyn Schlitz, PhD;

- A study researching the impact of external Qi Gong on cancer cells: effects of dose and distance, testing the hypothesis that human gene expression responds to the effects of intentionality on the part of Qi Gong masters operating from a distance, by Garret Yount, PhD, and Chinese Academy of Medical Sciences, Beijing, China.[39]

These are in addition to the studies documented in the film *The Living Matrix*.

The rigorously scientific approach taken in all these studies has done much to bring the potential of transpersonal experience into the realm of Western scientific medicine.

Integration into the Western Medical Model

This research results and the continued success of these methods—both ancient and modern—have required that Western medicine explore their applicability in the treatment of physical distress and disease. Sadly, though, methods like herbs, acupuncture, homeopathy, massage, therapeutic and touch as healing methods have typically been portrayed by the medical establishment as at best methods for enhancing the patient's comfort. Their successes are often ascribed by Western-trained physicians to a placebo effect, suggesting that their only value is in the mental state the patient brings to them and that no real physiological changes occur.

With such dismissals, the corporations and institutions whose livelihoods depend on reductionist "scientific" allopathic healthcare tenaciously hold on to their power, and, in spite of public interest in letting the alternative approaches of these 21st-century medicine methods fully emerge, the established powers resist. As a result, use of these methods as therapies is limited to a few practitioners scattered across the continents.

Yet the world turns and changes, seeming to accelerate as the new era emerges, offering more complete and profound kinds of human experience and healthcare. So the Western model is changing. It's in the early stages of what Thomas Kuhn called "a scientific revolution," in which one set of fundamental assumptions, which he called a "paradigm," is being replaced by another, radically different one.[40]

So, though scattered, the use of these methods is growing exponentially. Schools and colleges of Oriental, Homeopathic, and Natural Medicine are proliferating across the Americas and Europe, with curricula that include interpretation of energies as well as physical pulses and other symptoms. At the same time increasing numbers of practitioners and health organizations around the world are addressing the emotional and mental bases of the symptoms being displayed and are including energy-based healing methods like Reiki and Therapeutic Touch in their medical "toolkit."

ട

Meditation Methods Across Cultures

We can understand the effectiveness of meditation and other unified mind-body methods more easily when we step outside the framework of our normal, Western industrial culture's medical history and model. Because of the historical separation between the spiritual and the physical, we've tended not to see things the same way as people in many other cultures who've been quite effective healers for thousands of years. What follows is a brief summary of the history of meditation technuqes across human cultures.

Shamanic Traditions

The shamanic traditions are humanity's most ancient set of practices, deeply rooted in all Earth-centered cultures. Some have suggested that they may be part of the process by which self-consciousness emerged—possibly associated with the gazing into water and fire.[41] These are the practices of the wise ones, those who have separated themselves from the normal life of village or tribe to master their own emotions and physical responses and to develop the capacity to expand their awareness beyond their bodies and use their will for the good of their communities.

The men and women who have been so singled out are called "shamans" by anthropologists, because the first well-documented experience of these practices was in a Siberian tribe that called such a practitioner *saman*, a term that implies climbing a ladder. Shamans use a variety of disciplines to accomplish their goals, and many of their practices continue today, both in the "primitive" tribes of out-of-the-way places and in the "civilized" religious rites of both Eastern and Western traditions.

Michael Harner's *The Way of the Shaman*—both the book and the follow-up workshops and trainings—brought the essential concepts of shamanic traditions into Western culture. Doing so, he provided a context for such popular writings as those of Carlos Castaneda and Lynn Andrews. Since then, numerous books have been printed and studies completed exploring the nature and effectiveness of shamanic practices.

Nonetheless, Mircea Eliade's classic, *Shamanism: Archaic Techniques of Ecstasy*, written in the 1950s, remains the essential synthesis of the anthropological literature on the subject. Looking across cultures, he saw consistent patterns, chief among them being trance states in which the soul was believed to leave the body and travel to other worlds, often by means of a perceived ladder or staircase, and the use of secret languages, taught by spirits who travel on the ladder. These elements, he suggested, may contribute to the effectiveness of shamans as healers and prophets in their communities.[42]

The fact that there are consistencies across cultures in both principles and practice shouldn't be too surprising, because effective methods simply work, wherever they are applied. Among the specific practices common across shamanic traditions are the following:

- turning off "normal" thought processes to become silent inside, then listening to the body and the environment
- learning to manage the sensations and activities of the body
- study of the culture's traditions that explain how the world works and how people's minds, bodies, and communities function and develop
- study of one's own thought processes, dreams, and imaginations
- use of specific movements and sounds to enhance awareness, physical strength and agility, and overall wellbeing
- perceptual training to learn to "see" and "feel" energy shifts in the body and the community
- use of various movements, mental discipline, substances, and other methods for achieving altered states of consciousness in which awareness moves beyond the range of normal senses, space, and time.

These practices may be found among the Maori of New Zealand and the Eskimos of Alaska, among the hill tribes of Southeast Asia and the "witches" of Bulgaria, among the indigenous tribes of North America as well as those of the Amazon and Congo. They are also found woven into Buddhist, Taoist, and Hindu temple communities (as, for example, the Tibetan oracles that support the Dalai Lama), and in mystical Christian, Muslim, and Jewish communities, where ritual movement, physical austerities, and rhythmic chanting help to induce trance states, and they are the essence of the Sufi tradition.

Each culture has its own specific training protocols, disciplines, and expectations for these practices. Each culture has particular understandings of the nature of the shamanic experience, based on that culture's understanding of the nature of the world. Fundamentally, however, they achieve the same end, the enhancement of the individual's capacity to:

- "see" the world in terms of the energy patterns that compose our material experience,
- "hear" thoughts and sound patterns that affect the individual and community seeking assistance,
- act on the mind-body system of individuals in the community in a way that restores balance and harmony to the individual and the community as a whole, and
- perceive outside of normal space and time to forecast or prophesy important shifts and changes that affect the well-being of the community.

Judeo-Christian Mystic Healing Traditions

Christianity

Christianity is largely based on the capacity of one more-than-human person, called Jesus Christ, to heal others through touch and the spoken word—and his directive to his very human disciples to go out and do the same.

Descriptions of the early churches—in the Bible and other sources—always include people healing each other through prayer and laying on of hands. The apostle to the Gentiles, Paul, includes healing and prophesying among the gifts of the Spirit that come with becoming a Christian, and gives some guidelines for developing the capacity to do so. Peter, John, and others are reported by Luke to have effected healings by laying on hands, by declaration, and also when their shadows crossed the sick people who were laid out along the streets where they walked.[43]

The expectation of healing as part of being Christian was lost to the public and church congregations for centuries, until the emergence of "sacred relics" as vehicles for miraculous powers in the Middle Ages. Then, from the 11th century forward, pious Christians could go to a chapel or cathedral and touch, or simply view, a bit of bone or cloth they believed to be associated with a saint or holy person, and they'd often feel whatever pain or symptom that had troubled them fall away. The belief and expectation were enhanced by the presence of crutches, bandages, slings, and other prosthetic devices left behind by those who had gone away healed. This tradition remains alive today only in little-known but well-attended shrines that are scattered across the planet.

In convents and monasteries, however, expectation of miraculous events remained alive well into the 20th century. Stories of nuns and monks in ecstatic trance levitating, healing others through prayer or touch, living only on water or on the communion offered at daily Mass, and seeing profoundly moving visions of Jesus, his mother, and various saints, have circulated throughout the cloistered orders for centuries—and still do.

One famous set of stories concerns an Italian monk, Padre Pio. Many anecdotes describing his capacities are told, ranging from his stigmata to his levitations, which have been documented. Several books and websites tell of World War II pilots, sent to bomb an Italian village, turning back because a monk seemed to be floating in the air above it, indicating that they should go elsewhere. Most go on to say that the pilot or crew later saw pictures of, or met, the man— while witnesses in the monastery below observed the good monk praying in his cell that God and Mother Mary would protect the village. [44] Thousands of others report healings from his touch or word—and a few claim to have seen him in hospitals in other countries while he was observed to be in his monastery.

These stories, and the new interest in the Bible made possible by the reforms of the Vatican II Council of Bishops, inspired the birth of the charismatic movement within the Catholic Church during the 1960s and '70s. This movement, similar in many ways to that found in isolated American Pentecostal churches, has since expanded into mainstream Protestantism, where it has joined with the Pentecostal revivalist traditions of ecstatic trances and "faith healing" as one of many available modes of healing for the faithful.

Modern priests such as Ron Roth have joined Pentecostal ministers in touching people or speaking a few words and watching the infirm get up and walk away.[45] In both the Catholic and Protestant traditions, these clerics have felt what they call the Holy Spirit guiding them to say things and do things in church services that have led to the remission of cancers and other "terminal" illnesses among members of their congregations. For these Christians, the revival has moved from the tent to the sanctuary.

Judaism

Such miracles are not confined to Christian monks and mystics. Jesus was, after all, a Nazarene, dedicated to God in the Temple at Jerusalem and preaching in the synagogues around Judea and Galilee, as well as in the Temple itself. His healing miracles, the Jewish Talmud and other histories of the period tell us, were hardly unique. Many wandering preachers performed similar healings—perhaps best known of whom was Rabbi Ben Hillel. Simon bar Simeon (also known as Simon Magus) was another, who, according to the 1st-century Jewish historian Josephus, traveled to Rome in the years following Jesus' crucifixion and performed many similar miracles there. A cursory look at the Old Testament, particularly the stories of Elijah and Elisha, makes it clear that healing the sick, raising the dead, and prophesying the consequences of current actions were expected of one who had dedicated himself to God.

In modern Judaism, these kinds of experiences become possible for those who study the *Qabalah*, the mystery tradition based on a map of consciousness called The Tree of Life. Only men "over 40 and with a full belly" are encouraged to study *Qabalah*. It involves complex numerology and other symbolism as means of focusing attention, stilling the mind of its normal thought patterns, and allowing the awareness of a "still small voice," that of *Shekinah*, the wisdom that is the feminine aspect of the divinity. Having accomplished this mind stilling, the practitioner becomes empowered—as a healer and a prophet, for the good of his family and his community.

> There are many ways of using the *Qabalah* for healing... The Tree of Life, being a map of the whole person, is an ideal model to use for healing, whether of ourselves or others. A "whole healing" of any individual will include the whole Tree of Life— body, personality, soul and Spirit. For the healing to be effective it

will also include the relationship of the individual with their external world... on many levels, from the physical, through the psychological, to the deepest levels of spiritual connection... using the Tree as a healer of energy disorders and imbalances... it is undoubtedly true that we need to be clear vessels for the reception and transmission of the energies engendered by such work.[46]

Christian Science & New Thought

Another tradition deriving from Judeo-Christian roots was originally called Christian Science and has since split into two groups: the Church of Christ, Scientist, commonly called Christian Science, and the various organizations that make up what is known as the New Thought movement—including Science of Mind, Unity, Divine Science, and the Homes of Truth. These two groups are based on the ideas and practices of two mid-19th-century Americans: the philosopher Ralph Waldo Emerson and the healer in Maine we talked about earlier, Phineas Parkhurst Quimby.

Quimby had remarkable success relieving people of their symptoms by learning to still his mind and "go within" to discover the cause of their symptoms and help them change the belief systems that he found to be associated with those causes. Documented to have healed several thousand people in his offices in Belfast, Maine, Quimby believed he had discovered the method used by Jesus Christ. He felt that it was possible for anyone to learn the process, and taught it to whomever would take the time to study with him.

One of his patients and students, an itinerant homeopathic physician named Mary Baker Patterson, taught his method for several years and developed her own version of them following his death, describing them in her classic text, *Science and Health with Key to the Scriptures*. In 1875 she set up a small school in Lynn, Massachusetts. There she taught her method in a series of 6 lessons. She later married one of her students, Asa Eddy, and with him founded a school in Boston that a few years later became the Christian Science Church. They rapidly accrued thousands of members, building the grand "Mother Church," now a major Boston landmark, in 1903. Millions of people have been part of the Christian Science church during the 20th century, most of whom have used Eddy's methods of prayer and contemplation to heal themselves and others of various kinds of symptoms.

Perhaps the best known of her followers is Joel Goldsmith, who was a world famous healer and teacher during the mid-20th century and went on from Eddy's teachings to found an organization called The Infinite Way. His books, *A Parenthesis in Eternity, Consciousness Unfolding,* and *Practicing the Presence,* along with his volumes of Letters and recorded lectures, have provided thousands with support as they seek a way through the confusion of this passing Age of Anxiety:

> **Never forget this: The world, as a human world, is not the real world. There is nothing that we should or can do about the human situation. It is all a question of unfoldment. There must be a transcendental working out of all errors [in thinking]. To do that we turn within... We are to lift thought up out of its material sense and bring to light a spiritual awakening.**[47]

One of Mrs. Eddy's early students, Emma Curtis Hopkins, was a high school teacher with a lifelong interest in classical philosophy whose family was healed of a respiratory illness by one of Eddy's students. Hopkins found Mrs. Eddy's system to be limited and not entirely coherent, she set up her own school in Chicago. There she offered a slightly different version of the methods, later published in the text *Scientific Christian Mental Practice.* Though expressly Christian in orientation, Hopkins drew heavily on Eastern, Judaic, and classical writings to show the universality of the principles and practices she taught. Her lectures were often transcribed and later turned into books. In one of them, *Esoteric Philosophy,* she says:

> **When a man is sick, his mind causes the sickness. When you saw him sick, your mind saw his mind's opinion. If you rally your confidence to strike off the chains of his sickness, you are only engaging in a mental fight with him that one of you who is strongest will win.**
>
> **But who is That standing back of you both that never sees chains? Does That Mind know anything at all of illness?**
>
> **So the divisions of mind into mortal and immortal have been made. The mortal mind sees and talks of sickness.... It formulates all deformities, all ugliness. It sometimes formulates beautiful objects, but it is never the central fire. It is never the Mind that... stands back of mortal mind and shines through the chains.**[48]

Through her school Hopkins is documented as having healed, and in the process trained, thousands of people to work as healers and teachers. She did so by helping them see that their physical symptoms were direct results of their thoughts and feelings and showing them a series of steps to move beyond the old thinking to undo the cause of the symptoms. Her once infirm students included the founders of the Unity Institute (Myrtle Fillmore had been dying from TB and Charles Fillmore had a lame leg from childhood that was restored), the Homes of Truth (the Rix sisters had both been diagnosed with "untreatable" conditions), and the college of Divine Science (Nona Brooks was healed of throat cancer by a student of Emma's who'd been healed of uterine cancer). All of these individuals lived long, productive lives, and their teaching organizations were later expanded to include churches.

In 1906 Hopkins closed her school, then worked individually around the country for another two decades, writing and teaching people how to heal themselves by going within. Her *High Mysticism*, completed after the end of World War I, remains a classic guide to the integration of religious traditions into one clear path to the experience of the All as infinite wellbeing. In her last year of work she taught Ernest Holmes, who went on to found the Institute of Religious Science (now expanded into hundreds of Centers for Spiritual Living). Students of her students include Florence Scovel Shinn (author of *The Game of Life and How to Play It*), Emmet Fox (a contributor to the first AA program whose Wednesday evening lectures filled Madison Square Garden in the 1930s), Catherine Ponder and Eric Butterworth (both of whom redefined economics and restored prosperity to thousands with their versions of Hopkins' methods), and the modern healer and publisher Louise Hay—to name a few of the better known New Thought teachers, healers, and writers.

These traditions, derived from the works of Emerson and Quimby, have several things in common, based on their originators' experiences with healing and with maintaining health and prosperity:

- They assume that illness and all forms of individual distress are products of the workings of one's thoughts and feelings.
- They encourage the negation and release of thoughts and ideas that lead to illness and distress, replacing them with

affirmations of thoughts and ideas supporting health and well-being.
- They accept the possibility that one person can affect the mind-body of another simply with thought and words, and
- They emphasize the need to frequently "go within" (meditate, pray) to discover a deeper Truth or Reality in any situation.[49]

The Science of Mind, written by Ernest Holmes in 1925, following his series of lessons with Hopkins, is perhaps the best known work describing the essence of New Thought principles and practices. In it, he states:

> "It shall be as you believe." ...There is nothing in the universal order that denies the individual's good, or self-expression, as long as such self-expression does not contradict the general good.... Within us [therefore] is the possibility of limitless experience... The work is effective because the law is always in operation.[50]

Today, millions of people around the world use these basic principles and rely on the services of thousands of teachers and practitioners from these schools and churches, with many documented healings—of body, mind, economy, and relationships — occurring each year in each church or center.

Millions more follow a version of these principles as adapted by Louise Hay and presented in her very popular book, *You Can Heal Your Life*, with its index to symptoms and related beliefs, also published as *Heal Your Body*. Her experience helping thousands of AIDS patients avoid or long postpone the "automatic death sentence" they'd been told they were handed with their diagnosis attracted worldwide attention in the late 1980s. Her use of the treatment process taught by Hopkins and Holmes has helped her overcome her own "death sentence" of cancer, as well.

While often couched in the Christian terms that dominate American culture, both the method and the belief system underlying it are taught as drawing on the mystical traditions of the world, and often include teachings from other sacred scriptures. Although purely American in origin, they are, like the country, a "melting pot" of ideas and practices applied to enhance the wellbeing of both the practitioner and the client.

Hindu Mystic Healing Traditions

Yoga: Well-Being Through Union

Much of the early research on meditation and its effects involved the thousands of yogis who live in India. Westerners have long been fascinated by the range of skills and capacities demonstrated by long term practitioners of this ancient science. Reports of remarkable feats of control over the body, coupled with the sometimes overwhelming charisma of the more famous masters, fueled curiosity and concern.

While most Westerners think of the postures associated with *hatha yoga*, there are at least eight different yogas, each focusing on a different aspect of human development. Some of these are: *bhakti yoga*, the path of devotion; *prana yoga*, the mastery of energy flows through the breath; *karma yoga*, the path of action in the world; *raja yoga*, mastery of the whole self through the path of reason and intellect; and *tantra yoga*, mastery of the body through disciplined sensory experience. Each of these disciplines has been followed and taught by students and masters for millennia. Each of them has a whole unique set of principles and practices—and several different "schools" or approaches, with variations on those principles and practices—taught by different lineages of teachers.

It would be fair to say that the several yogas are prehistoric practices, handed down through generations of priests and teachers in the Vedic traditions that are now known, collectively, as Hinduism.

References to these practices may be found in the oldest known religious texts, called the *Vedas*, written in the root Indo-European language, Sanskrit, some 3500 years ago, based on oral traditions that go back another 3000 years. Many of the fundamental principles may be found in one small portion of those manuscripts, a sacred Hindu text called the *Bhagavad Gita*. It's the story of a young man's encounter with divinity—in the form of Krishna (sometimes called "the Hindu Christ")—and the many lessons that divine being imparts to him about the nature of the universe and how we can most effectively accomplish our life's goal of union with the divine.

The ancient word *yoga* is commonly translated as "union" and is the root of the English word "yoke." It's defined in the Gita as "the breaking of contact with pain." In practice, yoga is a path—often

Meditation Methods Across Cultures

described as a shortcut —to the continuous experience of nonlocal, nonattached awareness. This awareness is also considered a form of liberation, called, in Sanskrit, *moksha*, or *samadhi*. "The Atman [Real Self] shines forth in its own pristine nature, as pure consciousness."[51] All the practice, all the principles, and all the variations of yoga are designed to achieve this one end.

Along the way, yoga practices help the practitioner be healthier, happier, and more effective. Section One of the Yoga Sutras attributed to the great Hindu saint Patanjali in the 3rd century B.C.E. includes the following statements:

> #30. Sickness, mental laziness, doubt, lack of enthusiasm, sloth, craving for sense-pleasure, false perception, despair caused by failure to concentrate and unsteadiness in concentration: these distractions are the obstacles to knowledge.
>
> #31. These distractions are accompanied by grief, despondency, trembling of the body and irregular breathing.
>
> #32. They can be removed by the practice of concentration upon a single truth.[52]

The translators go on to say, "In order to achieve this concentration, we must calm and purify our minds,"[53] which, Patanjali tells us, may be done by changing our attitudes toward the people and events around us, and "The mind may also be calmed by [breathing] prana."[54]

Because of the enhanced capacities that come with the concentration required in the various yogas, many practitioners find themselves experiencing what, in our culture, are often called "paranormal" or "psychic" events. Patanjali says, in Section Three of his aphorisms, that, through such concentration, the mind:

> ...passes beyond the three kinds of changes which take place in subtle or gross matter and in the organs: change of form, change of time, and change of condition... one obtains knowledge of the past and the future... of what is subtle, hidden, and distant... of the constitution of the body... .[O]ne gains mastery of the elements... also perfection of the body, which is no longer subject to the obstructions of the elements... one gains mastery of the organs...[55]

One of the best known yoga practices in this country is the *kriya yoga* brought to the U.S. in the 1920s by Paramahansa Yogananda, founder of the Self-Realization Fellowship. He describes his method as follows:

> Kriya Yoga is a simple, psychophysiological method by which human blood is decarbonated and recharged with oxygen. The atoms of this extra oxygen are transmuted into life-current to rejuvenate the brain and spinal centers. By stopping the accumulation of veinous blood, the yogi is able to lessen or prevent the decay of tissues. The advanced yogi transmutes his cells into energy... uses his technique to saturate and feed his physical cells with undecayable light . . .[56]

As the most ancient documented set of mind-body practices, the yogas may be considered the first mind-body science. They provide the disciplined practitioner with the capacity to manage sensation, expand sensation beyond the body, overcome desire and attachment, along with the physical and emotional consequences of same, and exert influence on objects and events. They have been proved over and over, both within India and in Western scientific tradition.

Ayurveda

One of the many gifts Deepak Chopra has brought to Western healing practice is the native Indian system of healing known as Ayurveda (*Ayur* referring to "life" and *veda* meaning science"). In all of his books, and at his healing centers in Lancaster, Massachusetts and San Diego, California, Chopra has shown Westerners how healing can be accelerated through the combinations of diet, supplements, activity, meditation, and sound that make up the Ayurvedic approach. Though most Americans focus on the diet and supplements, Chopra emphasizes the role of meditation and sound in the practice. In *Quantum Healing* he describes their role and potential:

> In Ayurveda, bliss is the basis for three extremely powerful healing techniques. The first is meditation... Its importance is that it takes the mind out of its boundaries and exposes it to an unbounded state of consciousness. The other two... are... the Ayurvedic psycho-physiological technique... (we often prefer to use an informal name, the bliss technique)... [and]... primordial sound.[57]

Chopra tells us that these techniques move us beyond our normal way of thinking, stating that

> The bliss technique gives the patient the experience of himself as pure awareness, the ocean of wellbeing that is our basic prop and sustenance. With this technique alone it is possible to "drown" a disease in awareness and cure it... [58]

He points out that focused awareness, a shift in thought, can be enhanced through the use of sound:

> [T]o focus attention more precisely to heal... the primordial sound technique exists... With it, a specific tumor or arthritic joint can be attended to; a weak heart of clogged, arteries can be zeroed in on. You are not attacking the disorder with the primordial sound but paying closer attention to it—so close that the distortion of awareness lurking at the bottom of the disorder falls back into line... [59]

Awareness then, or focused attention, is the key. Chopra tells us that

> In Ayurveda, each and every symptom of disease, from a minor neck pain to a full-blown cancer, is under the control of attention... The Ayurvedic approach is to take a process already going on in the body and assist it naturally and without strain... Assuming that you are normally constituted, there is no innate reason why you cannot heal any disease with awareness.[60]

In this focus on awareness, Ayurveda relies on and embraces the yoga traditions of the Hindu culture in which it has emerged.

Tibetan Wisdom

It's probable that no nation in the 20th century was more completely destroyed than Tibet, and yet, marvelously, probably no other nation has been able to give more to the expanding paradigm of human potential. When China crushed defenseless Tibet in 1958 and 1959 there was a mass exodus of Tibetan people through the Himalayas into India—a dangerous exodus in which the Tibetans were hunted by the Chinese army and often overwhelmed by severe weather. Some estimate that only one out of 100 people succeeded in reaching India to survive, while many died of starvation and exhaustion in the process.

Remarkably, though, many of Tibet's greatest living Buddhist masters and doctors survived, protected by the people they led. They carried into India and from there into the West their knowledge of human psychology and potential, and higher orders of training, which had been kept alive for centuries in their remote mountain monasteries, temples, and villages.

Tibet has much to offer the world in the area of healing and medicine because of extraordinary events beginning in the first half of the seventh century, during the time of King Strongtsan Gampo. All around Tibet were nations—India, China, Nepal, Afghanistan, and Kashmir—in which Buddhist teachings were flourishing alongside traditional belief systems. Gampo was drawn to the teachings, converted to Buddhism, and began to bring Buddhist books into Tibet. Up till that time, there had been no written Tibetan language, but under his guidance, one was derived from Sanskrit and Pali for this purpose.

Srongstan Gampo also sought to strengthen Tibet's medical resources. "In pursuit of medical knowledge, the king held the first international medical conference in Tibet. Doctors came from India, Persia, and China."[61] Each of the doctors worked with a Tibetan who'd been trained in their language to translate one of their essential medical texts into Tibetan. The Persian medical system incorporated the ancient Greek medical system, which is the basis of Western medicine.

> The visiting Persian doctor, Galenos, was asked to remain in Tibet as the court physician. He married and had three sons, all of whom began separate medical family lineages.[62]

So the ancient medical knowledge of Western culture was kept alive continuity in Tibet.

Following Gampo, during the reign of King Trisong Detsen, there was a further major development in the history of Tibetan knowledge. In 749 he sent envoys to invite Padmasambhava, a widely renowned Buddhist master, to bring Buddhist wisdom and power into Tibet.

Padmasambhava was concerned for the future. In his homeland of Uddiyana, presently Afghanistan, where the Vajrayana Buddhist teachings had arisen, and in Ghandhara, south of Uddiyana, once a great center of Buddhism, great devastation had been caused by invading Huns. Thousands of Buddhist shrines, monasteries and temples had been desecrated.

In Buddhism, spiritual knowledge and medical knowledge were and are considered inseparable, and Padmasambhava saw that the Buddhist teachings and much of ancient wisdom, including profound medical knowledge, could be preserved in the mountain stronghold of Tibet for the future.[63] So he left to meet Trisong Detsun's envoys, whom he knew were coming to find him.

What happened next is one of the great events of human history and is remarkably well documented.[64] The combination of Padmasambhava's spiritual, and King Trisong Detsen's royal, power and grace was able to bring into Tibet not only essential collections of Buddhist scriptures from all Buddhist schools, but the texts and living embodiments of almost all sources of ancient wisdom, including medicine, astrology, mathematics, and other revered ancient sciences. They were able to bring in sacred texts of Indian Ayurvedic medicine and doctors who embodied that knowledge, the revered texts of Chinese medicine and doctors who embodied that knowledge, and more medical wisdom from Kashmir, Mongolia, Nepal, Sinkiang, Afghanistan, and Persia.

For over 20 years they assembled to translate and transmit this treasury of ancient wisdom. The translations were so carefully made that today some of them are being translated back into their original languages to replace lost libraries.[65]

> By the thirteenth century the Moslems had swept over the Indian regions and utterly destroyed all traces of Buddhist religion, culture, and learning... This meant ...Tibetans could no longer go to India for teachings, but this was not so important since they had already brought almost all spiritual and scientific lineages back to Tibet as living initiated lineages."[66]

That assembled treasury of knowledge became the basis for training in medicine as well as in the meditation sciences of Buddhism in Tibet—a system of training that lasted into the twentieth century.

Then, because of the Chinese invasion, this system was forced to come out of Tibet and into the world. So, starting in the 1960s, Tibetan Buddhist teachers and doctors came into Cold War Europe and the US, a world of vast military arsenals and economic pressures, and the associated stresses of the Age of Anxiety. And, because of their history, these teachers and doctors were able to provide powerful methods that can restore sanity and maintain health in times of great challenge.

Three Forms and Sources of Medical Wisdom in Tibet

We can identify three forms of training within the complexity of Tibetan medicine, and three sources of wisdom as it has been applied over the past thousand years.

The first form, traditional Tibetan medicine, is an integration of Chinese, Ayurvedic, and other medical systems brought into Tibet from the seventh century onwards, with its own distinctive characteristics. With the basic requirement of a compassionate nature and a good intelligence, through a training of more than ten years, the student learns the medicinal properties of thousands of plants and various other natural substances selected and compounded to produce sophisticated medicines, and acquired knowledge of the short- and long-term effects of the medicines. (Recently, Western pharmaceutical corporations have turned to these practitioners, along with indigenous healers around the world, having discovered the effectiveness of these medicines.) Training in human psychology and its relation to disease conditions is considered an essential basis for diagnosis and treatment. Medical capabilities included surgery, childbirth, near-death care, and after-death care. This is the form documented in the film *Tibetan Medicine, Buddhist Approach to Healing* and in *The Knowledge of Healing*, a film about the Dalai Lama's doctor and his methods.

The second form of Tibetan medical wisdom is the doctors who are also highly trained lamas, or meditation masters. According to the tradition, it's possible for someone with a high level of skill in both fields to carry their profound spiritual/psychological capability and extensive medical knowledge through the between-lives experience into the next life-time. This process of identifying the current incarnation of a previously honored teacher is illustrated in the film *The Little Buddha* and documented in the film *Unmistaken Child*. Dr. Trogawa Rinpoche, who has visited the West several times since 1982, represents this form of Tibetan medical expertise. In accordance with Buddhist tradition, he was highly regarded in his past incarnation as both a doctor and a consciously reincarnated spiritual teacher of the highest order. Now, as Trogawa *Rinpoche*, he has been trained from the youngest age to bring that endowment to an even higher level of capability and realization.

The third form of Tibetan medical wisdom is found in what is called, in Tibetan, *terma*, meaning "hidden treasure." These rare forms of knowledge were concealed by Padmasambhava throughout Tibet in the eighth century: in the earth, in works of art, and also in the unconditioned minds of his close disciples, to be carried through to future incarnations. The discovery of many of these hidden treasures and the utilization of their transmissions have been described in Tulku Thondup's *Hidden Teachings of Tibet*. However, the nature and utilization of medical *termas* is rarely disclosed, and then only through direct transmission, so is unpublished.[67]

Padmasambhava defined in the eighth century more than 350 disease conditions that would be mostly undiagnosed or wrongly diagnosed in our current era. As his biographer Yeshe Tsogyal recorded, some of his medical *termas* contain explicit instructions for psychological and medical treatments of AIDS and other "modern" conditions.[68] A few surviving Tibetan lamas, such as Shenphen Dawa *Rinpoche*, are believed to be reincarnated *tertons*, doctors who can utilize medical termas. How fully such knowledge will be utilized, preserved, developed, and passed on to future generations remains to be seen.

Three Sets of Teachings & Three Methods

Buddhism is a science of human development, not a religion. It is psychological and practical. The Buddha is not worshiped, but honored for having presented humanity with a great science of human development. He taught on ordinary and nonordinary levels for fifty years and revealed three distinct stages of evolutionary training, which evolved into three major Buddhist schools: *Hinayana, Mahayana,* and *Vajrayana*.

The Vajrayana Buddhism that is practiced in Tibet includes the Hinayana and Mahayana teachings and transmissions and may be the most complete system of human development available on our planet. It's characterized by a range of methods appropriate for the whole spectrum of human psychological types and levels. It offers a sophisticated description of human problems and the basis of disease conditions, as well as the potentials obstructed by those problems and conditions.

Ancient Wisdom, New Possibilities for Healing

Through the centuries and around the world, people have discovered and practiced a variety of mind-based methods with profound healing potential. Today, with our panoramic knowledge of human history and cultures, we are able to observe and select from a treasury of proven methods and understandings of profound value to human healthcare.

ಶ

Meditation In The United States

America has always welcomed people devoted to different religions and spiritual practices—as has been seen even among the First Peoples who populated the continent. Then, early decades of the colonial era saw the arrival of members of various Protestant sects, and the late 1800s brought in large numbers of Roman Catholic Christians from across Europe. The German Holocaust led to an influx of Jewish refugees in the 1940s. Then, in the 1960s and '70s, as noted above, Tibetan monks and masters found their way to these shores. Through the 1970s and '80s, Hindu teachers of various yoga practices were well received across the country. And, in the '90s, Sufi teachers began to offer mystical Islam, as well. Each of these traditions has brought a set of spiritual practices that contribute to our wellbeing as a population.

Meditation Is Established in American Culture

Explicit meditation practices were first made visible outside of the homes of individual practitioners in 1950, when D. T. Suzuki, a Japanese Zen Buddhist master, came to the U.S., settled in New York, and slowly helped establish Zen meditation in America. The Japanese word *Zen* means meditation, the "psychological method."

Then, quietly, like light entering a dark chemical process and changing it irreversibly, the recognition of inner light slowly emerged in Western society, through the 1970s and 1980s, during the advent of AIDS and amid the still unreleased stress of persistent thermonuclear threat. Both the lay public and medical professionals discovered that Buddhist meditation methods worked as a natural, healthy response to many health challenges.

By 1970, Suzuki and Chogyam Trungpa *Rinpoche*,[69] a Tibetan Vajrayana Buddhist master, were very visibly teaching meditation in various American cities, coast to coast. Maharishi Mahesh Yogi's Hindu-based Transcendental Meditation (TM) was introduced across the country shortly thereafter. Then Dudjom *Rinpoche*, head of the *Nyingma* lineage[70] of Tibetan Buddhism and a meditation teacher to the Dalai Lama, founded a center in New York City in 1976.[71] Since then there has been an exponential increase in the number of meditation centers in America, of every denomination.

Among the various forms of meditation in use in the West since that time, two forms have been most widely used: mindfulness meditation methods based on a Hindu-Buddhist practice called Vipashyana, and TM. Vipashyana (sometimes spelled Vipassana) is a silent psychological method in which attention is shifted from mind to awareness, slowing breathing down, which provides significant psychological and biological benefits. TM is a mantra-based technique in which the practitioner focuses attention on the repetition of a Sanskrit word or phrase. Both shift attention away from the disorder of the mind into a new state of consciousness, free of ordinary limitations, calming physiological processes.

Mindfulness Meditation

Mindfulness meditation is a psychological method based on an essential recognition of the difference between mind and awareness. This distinction is practical, definite, and transformative. It is readily understood by an increasing number of people as a useful, even essential, method for health and personal development.

Practitioners are able to recognize that their attention is usually lost in the uncontrolled activity of the mind, but they are readily able to shift their attention out of the chaos of the mind into stable open awareness, distinctly free of the mind.

Mindfulness is a process of seeing and appreciating how things work within the mind. One psychodynamic mechanism by which mindfulness seems to work is by helping the patient to distinguish primary sensory experience (for example, chronic pain, or physical symptoms of anxiety) from the secondary emotional or cognitive processes created in reaction to the primary experience.

It's been hypothesized that these secondary processes, when unrecognized, contribute greatly to a patient's distress and that, in the state of enhanced awareness, one is able to distinguish between the sensation itself and the suffering that the mind creates in response to the sensation.[72] Thus, mindfulness of pain allows one to separate the sensation from the suffering, which in turn tends to reduce anxiety and any tensions that might otherwise contribute to the pain.

Mindfulness is a calming process of concentration on breathing and flexibility of attention, simultaneously. It neither suppresses nor acts out emotions, but is a free middle path. Even though it is considered an ideal antidote to anxiety and stress, it is a new way of being rather than an antidote to mind and emotion. For awareness-based meditation, anxiety, impatience, and boredom are all good states to work with.

"Becoming aware is a human act that is so basic that it is independent of the contexts in which one becomes aware of one's own conscious activity."[73] Awareness, in most sacred traditions, is known to be primordially free of mind. It is the basis of human freedom and realization, free in the very contexts of suffering and sickness that mind may find itself lost in. Present-moment awareness, free of mind's anxieties about past and future, is the basis of calming and insight (which is the meaning of the words *Shamatha* and *Vipashyana*).

Mindfulness meditation is a method that offers a direct path to aware recognition of the time-based conditions of one's life. This recognition faces time and condition but is timeless and free of condition. The more that people practice the shift from anxious mind (bound by time) to awareness (timeless and open), the more they slow down their experience of time. The more that people shift from the experience of time to the experience of timelessness, the more they tend to experience "time stop." In the non-doing of mindfulness meditation, with its intentional giving up of involvement in time, people feel the boundless energy of the timeless and deathless state; they experience unconditioned immortal awareness. They move into a state of consciousness that is free of time, which, according to Tibetan understanding, is the basis of all healing.

Mindfulness meditation methods are readily accessible to most people. As a result, around the world today, millions of people are willingly giving up their habits of hope and fear to practice freedom from time, to experience the presence of unobstructed life, which is the heart of mindfulness meditation in its different forms.

The Sitting Practice of Mindfulness

Mindfulness meditation methods are simple and elegant. First there is attention to posture. Though there are profound reclining meditations (for example, the Progressive Relaxation body scan), sitting meditation, *dhyana asana,* is the perennial and prevalent mode of meditation. Many people initially have trouble sitting in a relaxed cross-legged posture, but most people can become at ease with some kind of sitting meditation. If you sit on the floor, it's best to use a cushion to lift your sacrum higher than your knees. If sitting on cushions or pillows or a meditation bench isn't possible, sitting in a chair is very good, especially if the participant can sit with the spine self-supporting, free of the back of the chair. If you can sit with the spine held upright as possible, effortlessly balanced, the spine will lift a little in a natural vertical alignment. This new balance will slow down and may stop unconscious tendencies of mind and body that support illness.

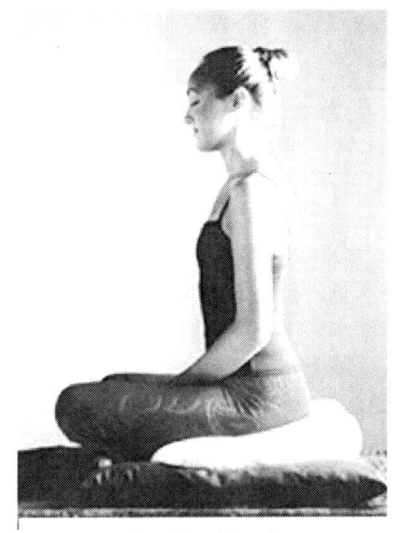

The ideal body position for all forms of mindfulness meditation.

To access self-reliance and deep potential, it helps to adopt an effortless upright posture, a kind of noble posture, with head, neck, and back aligned vertically. Such posture aligns a natural vertical flow of life force. If the spine is balanced, self-supporting, and if the head is balanced over that, the spine will tend to lift a little, releasing pressure on its vertebrae and nerves, which is conducive to healing and freedom.

Meditation posture can be the position of by which revolution is made possible. It can be a way of balancing the body "to stop the world." It can be an effortless way of sitting into potential, a way of directly sitting into life itself.

Sitting meditation lets you sit into stillpoint, which encourages the mind to break from its relentless activity. Sitting into stillpoint facilitates the natural shift from mind to awareness, a transformative shift, a revolutionary shift. Because sitting meditation is good for slowing down the mind, even stopping the mind, it has enabled people for centuries to access the healing return to awareness, to come back to the unlimited human potential.

Once seated, the breathing is the immediate concern. You raise the intention to breathe with awareness. You place attention on your breath. You patiently keep present and stay with your breath. Thinking forcefully takes you out of the present moment, preventing you from being present—until your awareness brings you back to your breath. Breath is body; body is present. The person who meditates this way keeps coming back to the breath to calm down the mind.

Coming back to awareness and breath counteracts the reactiveness and momentum of the mind. It starts to cut the force of the mind. With the method of awareness meditation one makes a "conscious effort to move in a direction of healing and inner peace. This means learning to work with the very stress and pain that is causing you to suffer."[74]

People use the practice of mindfulness meditation to directly engage awareness in the present moment. "We speak of the 'practice' of meditation, and the 'practice' of mindfulness, meaning the actual engagement in the discipline, the inward gesture that invites and embodies it."[75]

Mindfulness meditation practice has various forms, used for various periods of time, but its aim is to develop a continuity of awareness. The practice is a direct and proven path to unlimited inner resources and the source of awareness.[76]

Meditation Research

The science of mind-body medicine could be said to have been founded at the Harvard Medical School in the mid-19th century, through the world-famous work of Oliver Wendell Holmes, MD, and then William James, MD. In the 20th century their work was advanced by Walter Cannon, MD, and then by Herbert Benson, MD. Benson's renowned work in measuring the medical benefits of meditation, from the late 1960s to the present day, have defined the present field and science of mind-body medicine.

It's safe to say that no spiritual or healing practice from another culture or spiritual tradition has been studied so much in the West as meditation. From the work by William James in the mid-19th century to that of Benson and his lab director, Joan Borysenko MD, in the late 20th, we have thousands of documented experiments and longterm tracking results. The following pages give an overview of some of the highlights.

Early Research in Other Countries

Clearly, meditation and its use in healing is very old, deep in our human heritage. Its visible emergence in Western scientific cultures, however, has occurred only in the past 100 years. From the 1920s onward in India, at Lonavla near Bombay, there was a major center for meditation and medicine. Using a system of physical culture and yogic therapies for many afflictions, it had support from the governments of British India and England, the Indian Health Agency, and American foundations.

This yoga therapy center was also a research center. Its studies began a process ensuring that America would become an important center of mind-body medicine and meditation research.

Also in India, from the 1930s into the 1950s, dramatic demonstrations of the power of meditation over vital functions were documented. In each case there was a yogi who wanted to demonstrate for science a higher order of human function.[77]

One yogi was buried completely in a small concrete chamber, cut off from oxygen, with more than 10,000 people watching. The chamber was covered with wood and earth for eight days.

We frequently see television dramas illustrating how the ER trauma team works on people who have been oxygen deprived for even a few minutes. It's understood that without oxygen the brain will lose function and can die quickly. After a period of forty-five minutes to an hour of dramatic measures, including electric shock and stimulants, the doctors call it "time of death."

Amazingly, however, after an hour, the buried yogis were just beginning to get into their meditation demonstration. One came out after 2 days, stood, and then did handstands. The one who was completely buried for 8 days had gone from a heartrate of 50 beats per minute through a rapid drop-off to no perceptible heart beat after 29 hours of burial, where it remained until ½ hour before the previously agreed time he was to be removed. Then his heart resumed beating at 50 beats per minute. Apparently he had an internal clock running during his burial as well as an extraordinary control of his breath and his heart.[78]

The buried yogis mostly came out smiling. The Western scientists and journalists observing them wondered: "how did he live? What did he do?"

In the 1960s, two physicians at the University of Tokyo studied brainwave changes during meditation by Zen teachers and their disciples from the Soto and Rinzai Zen centers. Pulse rates, respiration, galvanic skin response, and electrical information were given by good-natured advanced and less advanced practitioners, who clearly saw that they could help science understand meditation. In these studies, four stages of meditation were observed, each measured in terms of the brainwave patterns that showed up on electroencephalograms (EEGs).

> Stage 1: Characterized by the appearance of alpha waves (the brain-wave pattern associated with dreaming, daydreaming, and being "in the zone").

> Stage 2: Increase in amplitude of persistent alpha waves (associated with a stronger sense of being "in the zone").

Stage 3: Decrease in alpha-wave frequency (associated with relaxation).

Stage 4: The appearance of rhythmical theta trains (the brainwave pattern associated with deep rest).

These findings indicate that Zen practice promotes a serene, alert awareness that is consistently responsive to both external and internal stimuli.[79]

Between 1970 and 1972, Herbert Benson, a cardiologist with strong mind-body medicine inclinations, went to Asia on several occasions to study the biology of adept Vajrayana (Tibetan) Buddhist practitioners. There he observed evidence of life-enhancement through control of vital processes. He was particularly impressed by the now famous *tummo,* known as "Wisdom Fire," practice. He observed several Buddhist yogis go out into a subzero Himalayan night wearing nothing but a cotton cloth. After sitting and developing the tummo heat, they were covered with wet sheets. They showed their Wisdom Fire capability by drying several sheets in one night. As a result of this and other experiences, Benson saw that meditation offered remarkable biological potential and went on to study various meditation methods, qualifying and quantifying these benefits for medical science.[80]

Meditation Research in the United States

Boston area hospitals have a heritage of being in the forefront of medical advances and the Buddhist teachers were interested in Western medicine. In 1979, Jon Kabat-Zinn established the Mindfulness-Based Stress Reduction (MBSR) clinic at the University of Massachusetts Medical Center (UMMC), the Boston area's fourth largest hospital. There, the successful use of Buddhist meditation in anxiety and pain management was established and made part of popular culture. In 1981, Herbert Benson established the Mind/Body Clinic of the Harvard Medical School at Boston Deaconess Hospital and there developed an Americanized approach to meditation that established the physiological processes involved in its effectiveness and brought the methods into popular use.

These two programs continue today as outstanding clinical and research programs exploring the medical uses of meditation. The

UMMC clinical program influenced the Harvard program and has been the model for hundreds of clinical programs in meditation in hospitals and medical centers throughout the United States and Canada. This kind of medicine doesn't have a lobby but it does have large public support and is the most proven of the "alternative" medicines. Of the thousands of people who have participated in the UMMC and Harvard Medical Center programs (more than 30,000 between the two of them), most have been under medical insurance coverage, which indicates some level of institutional support for this practical and clinically proven medical method. Also, many healthcare providers have attended the meditation-medicine programs, both to learn methods that could help their patients and for the sake of their own wellbeing.

The UMMC Research

Mindfulness meditation as presented at the UMMC is a form of *Vipashyana,* the "insight" meditation prevalent across India and Southeast Asia and based on 2,400 years of Buddhist tradition. UMMC has successfully applied mindfulness to reclining progressive relaxation (PR) as one of the integral methods of its program, using breathing as a key to pain management and symptom reduction.

The results achieved at the UMMC program are very impressive. From 1979 to this writing, more than 25,000 people are graduates of the program, most of them under medical insurance coverage, and most of them experiencing remarkable reductions in symptoms of a wide range of diseases, including cancer, AIDS, heart disease, diabetes, and anxiety disorder.

Jon Kabat-Zinn, the developer and original director of the UMMC program, has told the story of its development and given us a summary of its research observations in his book, *Full Catastrophe Living*. The practice that is the cornerstone of the program may be outlined as follows:

Step 1: Sit quietly in a comfortable position.

Step 2: Eyes may be open or closed.

Step 3: Relax your muscles.

Step 4: Keep your attention on your breath, being particularly attentive to the relaxing out-breath and the moment of gap or stillness before the next breath.

Step 5: Breathe slowly and naturally. Belly breathing is best: breathe down and calm down.

Step 6: Recognize your thoughts, the anxious movement of the mind. Return to open awareness. Return to calm. Keep returning to awareness. Keep calming down.

Step 7: Continue for ten to twenty minutes. Sit for a specific amount of time.

Step 8: Do not stand immediately. Continue sitting quietly for a minute or so, allowing other thoughts to return. Then sit for another minute before rising.

Step 9: Practice this technique once or twice daily.

With this and related methods, Kabat-Zinn observes symptom reduction and health development in a variety of major disease conditions, with patients reporting significant benefits in treating cancer, pain, and anxiety. He says that it clearly has the ability to bring its practitioners "to a new order of reality."[81]

The UMMC program continues to inspire people to meditate and to help themselves with their health problems. People participating in the UMMC program learn to calm their body and mind to find inner balance in the face of the challenging disturbances of life. The obvious benefits help people commit to keep meditation at the heart of their life. Shifts in certain heath-maintaining hormones have also been observed, which we will detail later.

The UMMC uses the classical mindfulness of breath as the basis of shifting from mind to awareness. Working with breathing is a key to all the UMMC program methods: sitting and reclining meditation, yoga, and walking meditation.

> The mind will challenge you to keep you from calm breathing, but people find that they can stay with deep breathing and calm down. If we follow the breath as a path, it has the power to help us balance body and mind.[82]

The Harvard Research

Herbert Benson has given us both research and a method at Harvard's Mind/Body Clinic, which he established in September 1981, with Joan Borysenko as director. Drawing on the commonalities across several of these meditation methods, Benson developed what he called "The Relaxation Response." Having spent years studying the medical uses of meditation, Benson determined that he had amassed

> significant evidence of the tremendous diversity of medical conditions that the elicitation [Relaxation Response] together with other self-care strategies... can heal or cure.[83]

The Benson method is similar to Kabat-Zinn's, as follows:

> Step 1: Pick a focus word or short phrase that's firmly rooted in your belief system.
>
> Step 2: Sit quietly in a comfortable position.
>
> Step 3: Close your eyes.
>
> Step 4: Relax your muscles.
>
> Step 5: Breathe slowly and naturally, and as you do, repeat your focus word, phrase, or prayer silently to yourself as you exhale.
>
> Step 6: Assume a passive attitude. Don't worry about how well you're doing. When other thoughts come to mind, simply say to yourself, "Oh well," and gently return to the repetition.
>
> Step 7: Continue for ten to twenty minutes.
>
> Step 8: Do not stand immediately. Continue sitting quietly for a minute or so, allowing other thoughts to return. Then open your eyes and sit for another minute before rising.
>
> Step 9: Practice this technique once or twice daily.

Benson proved that the practice of this simple but sound method improves biologic function by slowing the internal state. It lowers blood pressure, slows heart rate, and reduces oxygen consumption. It rests metabolic activity, leaving more oxygen available for other functions.

> As far as science knows, the calming effects of the relaxation response cannot be brought about as dramatically or as quickly by any other means.[84]

The Center's director, Joan Borysenko, observed some of the characteristics of those engaged in this meditation practice as follows:

> Breathing rate and oxygen consumption decline because of the profound decrease in the need for energy. Brain waves shift

from an alert beta-rhythm to a relaxed alpha-rhythm . . .Blood flow to the muscles decreases, and instead, blood is sent to the brain and skin, producing a feeling of warmth and rested mental alertness. It was by learning to induce the relaxation response that I began to reverse symptoms that were severe enough to send me to the emergency room. [85]

Specific gains they identified from the use of meditation can be considered in three categories:

- self-awareness and attention
- distinct physiological shifts
- energetic enhancement

Most long-term meditators or practitioners of the Relaxation Response have experienced benefits in one or all of these areas. Some of the more important medical benefits of meditation observed in Harvard's Mind/Body Clinic research include:

- Patients with hypertension experienced significant decreases in blood pressure and needed fewer or no medications over a 3-year measurement period.
- Patients with chronic pain experienced less severity of pain, more activity, less anxiety, less depression, and less anger, and they visited the managed care facility where they received care 36 percent less often in the two years after completing the program than they did prior to treatment.
- Patients with cancer and AIDS experienced decreased symptoms and better control of nausea and vomiting associated with chemotherapy.
- Patients who suffered from anxiety or mild or moderate depression were less anxious, depressed, angry, and hostile.
- Patients undergoing painful X-ray procedures experienced less anxiety and pain and needed 1/3 the amount of pain and anxiety medications usually required.
- Working people experienced reduced symptoms of depression, anxiety, and hostility and had remarkably fewer medical symptoms.
- Patients who had open-heart surgery had fewer post-operative cardiac arrhythmias and less anxiety following surgery.

Transcendental Meditation Research

Perhaps the most numerous studies of meditation and its benefits are those focusing on a simple meditation practice introduced in the United States in the late 1960s by the Hindu teacher, Maharishi Mahesh Yogi, called Transcendental Meditation (TM). Today more than 500 published articles, involving thousands of meditators, are abstracted on the TM website (www.tm.org), alone.

Though many observers doubt the objectivity of the TM researchers, Benson decided to make use of their work and further the research on TM. The first clinical research on the technique, conducted at UCLA and Harvard medical schools, was published from 1970 to 1972 in the respected journals *Science, American Journal of Physiology*, and *Scientific American*. These landmark studies revealed that the Transcendental Meditation technique produced a unique state of mind and body called "restful alertness." The mind settles down to its most silent level. Since the mind and body are intimately connected, as the mind settles down the body also settles down to a deep state of rest.

> Researchers discovered significant reductions in respiration, minute ventilation, tidal volume, and blood lactate, and significant increases in basal skin resistance. All of these physiological measures represent a state of deep relaxation, even deeper than sleep. And they found that even though the body is in a state of deep rest, the mind is alert rather than asleep, indicated by an increased abundance of alpha waves in the EEG... For the past 30 years, many other researchers have confirmed and expanded upon this initial research... the experience... is correlated with greater creativity, improved learning, higher IQ, better grades, higher moral reasoning, increased brainwave coherence, and improved neurological functioning of the body.[86]

The practice is simple:

Step 1. All TM students are given a unique *mantra*—a Sanskrit word or phrase—that is intended to assist them in releasing their particular pattern of thought and feeling.

Step 2. They are guided through a process of relaxing the body and repeating the mantra,

Meditation Research

> Step 3. They are then sent home to perform the practice for twenty minutes, morning and evening.

The initial training is sufficient for most, but it is possible to take advanced trainings, ultimately learning to train others. Students are encouraged to simply focus on repeating the mantra, silently, and to return to the mantra whenever they notice other thoughts or images. "Like bubbles of air in the ocean, simply watch any thoughts that bubble up as they go by, without letting them affect you," said Maharishi in one of his question-and-answer sessions.

Based on ongoing studies, the TM organization publishes the following list of benefits for people doing the practice:

- Clearer Thinking: Develop your full mental potential, improve your memory, enhance creativity, and sharpen your intellect.
- Better Health: Become more rested and relaxed, increase immunity to disease, reverse the effects of aging, and enjoy greater energy and vitality.
- More Fulfilling Relationships: Enjoy closer friendships, increased calmness, more self-confidence, and less anxiety and stress.
- A Peaceful World: Contribute your share to world peace by reducing your own stress level and radiating an influence of harmony to your surroundings.
- Personal Growth: Experience transcendental consciousness at the quietest level of your mind, and grow toward higher states of consciousness—enlightenment. [87]

The theory developed by TM researchers to explain these benefits is that, by focusing on repeating a properly selected mantra instead of one's normal thoughts, the mind becomes calmer and the mind-body system becomes more coherent in its functioning. In addition, the calmed mind begins to operate at a new level of consciousness, which they call "transcendental consciousness," that permits the meditator access to more stored memories and learned or observed skills than would otherwise be available.

Many of the published studies focus on the technique's clinical effects. Dr. Dean Ornish calls TM

> ...an ancient stress-management technique [that] may decrease blood vessel blockage and help people avoid a heart attack or stroke. A study published in the March 2000 issue of the journal Stroke shows that TM decreased the thickness of blood vessel walls, a known risk factor for stroke and heart disease. ...The researchers found that two 20-minute sessions of daily TM led to a widening of the space inside the practitioners' arteries. In the comparison group, which did leisure activities instead of TM, arterial thickening continued to worsen. [88]

Today, more than ten million people around the world have completed the initial TM training, with several thousand of them going on to advanced levels.

As the numbers increase, more research has been done on what is called "the Maharishi Effect," or the impact that a group of people meditating regularly has on the larger community. One study, described in the film *What the BLEEP Do We Know!*?* had 4,000 people meditating on a regular basis through the summer in Washington, D.C., during which period the rate of violent crime was reduced by a third. Another study, posted on the TM website, shows a marked decrease in global terrorist activity whenever a TM conference has been held.[89]

The Ornish Program

Dean Ornish, MD, a cardiologist, wished to enhance the ongoing well-being of his heart patients. Seeing the effectiveness of methods like RR and TM, he developed a medical meditation program using absorptive deep breathing, which is a beathirng of energy, which the Hindus call *prana*, from the universal field.

> In this system we inhale not only oxygen but also energy, or prana. In Sanskrit, prana means both breath and spirit. It is a universal energy in the air. In the West it's called vital energy and is known to be breathable.[90]

Dr. Ornish's program differs from the UMMC programs in the concern with deep breathing. He taught people to breathe deeply, to inhale vital encrgy in the air (called in Sanskrit, *prana*) and take it into their bodies.

Dr. Ornish comments on meditation:

Meditation is the practice and process of paying attention and focusing your awareness.. when you... concentrate any form of energy, including mental energy, you gain power. When you focus your mind, you concentrate better. When you concentrate better, you perform better—you can accomplish more... as you experience a profound state of relaxation, deeper even than sleep... blood pressure decreases, your heart rate slows, your arteries dilate, you think more clearly.

...you enjoy your senses more fully... Anything that you enjoy—food, sex, music, art, massage, and so on—is greatly enhanced by meditation... your mind quiets down and you experience an inner sense of peace, joy, and well-being... Before, I thought peace of mind came from getting and doing; now, I understand that it comes from being. It is our true nature to be peaceful until we disturb it.

Finally, you may directly experience and become more aware of the transcendent interconnectedness that already exists... Like peace, joy, and well-being.[91]

Through Dr. Ornish's holistic approach, including dietary changes, exercise, and guided meditation, many people with "terminal" cases of heart disease have seen significant results and much longer life spans than would be expected under more typical medical protocols. This success has led to an overall shift in the medical profession's treatment of heart conditions.

Psychological Benefits of Meditation

Summarizing research referred to in the above sections in their book, *The Physical and Psychological Effects of Meditation*, Murphy and Donovan describe increases in the following psychological capacities as benefits of meditation:

- perceptual ability
- concentration and intelligence
- empathy
- creativity
- self-actualization
- reaction time and physical motor skill[92]

They observe that various meditation schools offer methods to cultivate clarity, flexibility, efficiency, and a broadened range of psychological functions. This is seen in the meditation results reviewed in the 51 pages of research abstracts in their book. Though the above-indicated psychological benefits are important in maintaining a healthy human, with respect to pathological conditions the pain management potential of meditation makes it an invaluable resource for many areas of medicine.

Meditation and Pain Management

Extensive research conducted by Kabat-Zinn and others at UMMC demonstrated that meditation produced significant reductions in the following:

- present moment pain,
- negative body image,
- inhibition of activity (movement limitation),
- psychological disturbance,
- anxiety and depression, and
- the need for pain-related drugs. [93]

These benefits are considerably more complex than simply increased tolerance of pain, which was the accepted understanding prior to their work.

These results occur because, with the mindfulness meditation method used at UMMC, people learn to distinguish between mind and awareness. As people learn to expose mind to awareness, they learn to see how the mind dwells on anxiety and fear and burns up energy, making them exhausted, limiting their ability and reserves. They learn that they're capable of staying in the present moment, even while experiencing high levels of pain. They see that their mind likes to avoid being present by making a big deal about the pain, creating the experience of suffering. They see that for healthy reasons they want to stay in open awareness, free of their mind, and avoid their own creation of suffering.

People practicing mindfulness meditation see that they can develop fearlessness and gain energy by distinguishing between pain sensations and what the mind is trying to do with them. They avoid letting their mind agonize and waste energy reserves. They see that they have a choice to prevent distress and build courage and inner strength in the process. They learn that staying with present-moment pain naturally releases endorphins, the body's natural painkillers, which then increase the ability to stay present.

The more one is present with the sensation, the higher the endorphin levels and the greater the development of fearlessness. This heals those situations in which suffering weakens reserves. Mindfulness encourages an attitude that fosters health. With psychiatric and pain management drugs costing more than a hundred billion dollars a year, we have many reasons to ask medical science to advance the use of the medical art of meditation, for pain management and for greater health.

Meditation and Learning

A number of studies have been done over the years by Charles Tart at the University of California, researchers at the Maharishi Institute, Harvard, and the Massachusetts Institute of Technology (MIT) exploring the effects of regular meditation and brain development. Some of the most recent research was done under the direction of Catherine Kerr at MIT.

As published in the *Brain Research Bulletin* in April of 2011, the group found significant increases in Alpha brain wave patterns. Christopher Moore, one of the MIT neuroscientists performing the study says:

> These activity patterns are thought to minimize distractions, to diminish the likelihood stimuli will grab your attention. ... Our data indicate that meditation training makes you better at focusing, in part by allowing you to better regulate how things that arise will impact you.[94]

Eileen Luders of UCLA found that there was a deep connection between faster processing of information and years of meditation. Using neuro-imaging, Luders and her team found that meditation adds folds to the cerebral cortex, which plays a central role in memories, attention, thought and consciousness. The folding of the cortex stimulates mind processing, causing a boost in your memorizing skills, decision making, solving complex problems etc. In meditators with more than 20 years experience,, that can be as much as a tenfold increase.[95]

Physiological Benefits of Meditation

Extensive research has shown that significant biological problems are directly caused by anxiety and stress. In brief, anxiety causes an overproduction of the hormones adrenaline and cortisol, which suppress important biological functions, including the immune system, in order to shift energy into muscle systems for a "fight or flight" reaction, based on old instinctive tendencies.

Anxiety suppresses immune system function primarily through elevated levels of cortisol in the bloodstream. Anxiety and stress, with accompanying hormonal imbalance, have been proved, through extensive research, to be primary factors in the weakening of health and the cause of various immune-deficiency diseases.

The widespread chemical treatment of anxiety has resulted in additional biological and psychological problems.

In contrast, self-calming meditation has been shown to directly reduce adrenaline and cortisol secretion, naturally restoring hormonal balance in general and normalizing immune system function. In addition, meditation produces elevated levels of the major hormones melatonin, DHEA, and serotonin, and endorphins, powerful pain-relieving, pleasure-causing agents secreted by the nervous system. Benson speaks of the direct health and medical impact of meditation as follows:

> When you focus for a short time, gently brushing aside any intrusive thoughts, your mind and body suddenly become a five star resort in which all the service personnel make your restoration and health their priority and are especially concerned with alleviating the harmful effects of stress. This great team of stress-busters and body-relaxers emerge when everyday thoughts and worries are put aside.[96]

Benefits with respect to treatment of major disease conditions, including cardiovascular disease, cancer, and others, are described elsewhere in this book. Presently our focus will be primarily on three areas: hormonal balance, immune system enhancement, and management of pain and anxiety. These subjects are of fundamental concern to all biopsychic disorders.

Hormonal Balance - Melatonin

The fact that meditation produces elevated levels of melatonin, the hormone secreted by the pineal gland located at the center of the brain, was first disclosed by research conducted at UMMC.[97] The pineal gland has drawn the attention of human insight for a long time. In the 17th century René Descartes, in his famous *Treatise of Man*, called the pineal gland the seat of the human psyche, the principal location of self-awareness. Hundreds of sacred images include a pinecone as a symbol for the pineal. More than 3,500 years ago, the Hindu *Vedas* described the pineal gland in the context of the energy body:

> The [pineal] gland was portrayed as one of the seven chakras, or centers of vital energy, which are arranged along the central axis of the body. The pineal gland was thought to be the supreme or crown chakra . . . the ultimate center of spiritual force.[98]

While these insights are inspiring for people interested in meditation, the current worldwide interest in melatonin, evident in the presence of hundreds of research papers and books on the subject, is focused on its biological benefits, particularly concerning its remarkable effects on the human immune system. Melatonin many be the most potent and versatile of the antioxidants. It directly stimulates interleukin-2 activity that in turn stimulates the increase of all the various cells of the immune system, in a pervasive optimization of immune function, and directly restores and increases T-helper cell production in bone marrow. As a result, it has been used as a therapeutic agent in both cancer and AIDS therapy.

Melatonin is known to have a calming effect, bringing a sense of contentment and improved mood, and is often used as a sleep aid. Especially when produced naturally to elevated levels, it makes normal sleep and rest possible even in challenging situations.

Hormonal Balance - DHEA (dehydroepiandrosterone)

DHEA, produced in the adrenal glands just above the kidneys, is the most plentiful human hormone and is essential for health. Like melatonin, it tends to diminish in the body as people age. An increased level of life-enhancing DHEA in older meditation practitioners was one of the first biological benefits of meditation to be observed.

Like melatonin, DHEA has a variety of health-increasing benefits. It is an immunity enhancement agent that has been proved to be beneficial in the prevention and treatment of cancer, cardiovascular disease, diabetes, lupus, and other disorders. DHEA stimulates the production of monocytes (T-cells and B-cells), potent immunity biochemicals that cause the production of other immune system agents. T-cells are white blood cells produced in the bone marrow that produce two powerful immune system agents—interleukin-2 and gamma interferon—intelligent defense agents that help maintain health.

DHEA is good for the bones, muscles, blood pressure, vision, and hearing. It is the substance from which the male and female hormones are developed. It's probably the essential reason that kidney energy, called *chi,* is an important concern in Chinese medicine. DHEA contributes to vitality and youthfulness. It's a mood elevator that makes people feel and look better. It enhances brain biochemistry and growth. Anxiety and stress lower normal DHEA levels in the bloodstream, while meditation elevates DHEA levels.

Hormonal Balance - Endorphins

Meditation is also known to increase levels of endorphins, a set of peptides secreted throughout the nervous system that have very strong pain-relieving and pleasure-inducing effects, similar to morphine.

Of these powerful chemicals, the endocrinologist Deepak Chopra writes:

> Thus the brain [and nervous system in general] produces narcotics up to 200 times stronger than anything you can buy... with the added boon that our own pain-killers are nonaddictive. Morphine and endorphins both block pain by filling a certain receptor on the neuron and preventing other chemicals that carry the message of pain from coming in, without which there can be no sensation of pain, no matter how much physical provocation is present.[99]

The above four vital biological substances produced by meditation contribute to immune system strength and personal feelings of wellbeing, essential for disease prevention, recovery, and maintaining health. Many more such substances remain to be studied.

Meditation as a Means for Promoting Wellbeing

Kenneth Pelletier, MD, in *Mind as Healer/Mind as Slayer*, his excellent overview of mind-body medicine, describes meditation as "psychologically and physiologically more refreshing and energy restoring than sleep."[100] He defines two basic methods of meditation through which the practitioner may come to a psychological state called *satori*, or transcendent awareness:

> The object of both kinds of meditation methods, focusing of attention on an object of meditation, such as a mantra or a physiological process, such as breathing; and opening up of attention, such as in Zen or Vipashyana meditation, which use focus on the flow of the breath as a basis for staying open.[101]

The primary affect of meditation, Pelletier says, is to gain mastery over attention.[102] That is the key to a shift of function and direction in health. Awareness of mind, awareness of thought, awareness of anxiety is key to the quality of the Benson technique as it is of meditation in general.

The healing qualities of meditation documented across all the research include:

- Intervention: Meditation is well documented as an intervention reducing the effects of many conditions.
- Empowerment: Discipline empowers; commitment to an ongoing practice is essential; it enables people to develop inner resources, to be progressively less limited by conditioning, to touch upon the resource potential in the unconditioned state.
- Symptom Reduction: Meditation brings significant reductions in many medical and psychological symptoms; but in addition, people change for the better, which is healing, beyond body and mind.
- Enduring Effects: In the UMMC program the changes produced over eight weeks lasted up to three years without continuity of

the practices. However, 85 percent of the participants continue the practices.

- Behavioral Shifts: Meditation encourages conscious action. It keeps people out of emergency rooms and off mind-dulling addictive chemical agents as they take on new, consciously chosen behaviors.

Because of these qualities, meditation has been found to be useful in the treatment of a variety of chronic conditions, including asthma and fibromyalgia,[103] insomnia, migraine and cluster headaches, and infertility.[104]

The above characteristics of meditation are useful in what are usually considered terminal situations, as well. The American Medical Association website lists the major causes of death as follows:

- cardiovascular and heart disease (including stroke)
- cancer
- hospital care (in the form of adverse drug reactions and death from surgery)[105]

The research shows that meditation methods could well reduce these numbers.

Cardiovascular Care

Cardiovascular disease, especially stroke, is the greatest health concern in America and in the West in general. The dietary causes are well documented.[106] Concerning the psychological and emotional causes of cardiovascular problems, we know this: We don't usually respond to stressful situations physically, and because people don't burn up the energy released by the fight-or-flight reaction, they are vulnerable to various negative consequences.[107] Meditation is an antidote for cardiovascular problems as follows:

- Stress and anxiety call for greater blood flow, more forceful heart beats, and higher blood pressure. Meditation moderates heart beat and lowers blood pressure. Higher blood pressure strains and enlarges the heart. It also contributes to the blockage of the arteries, arteriosclerosis. The high blood pressure and blockages lead to the bursting of arteries, causing stroke and internal bleeding. Regular meditation can prevent and reverse heart disease.[108]

Meditation Research 69

- Adrenaline caused by anxiety and stress can disturb the heart rhythms, causing cardiac arrhythmias. Meditation balances heart beat irregularities.
- Anxiety and stress lower people's threshold of pain, which may cause other problems. Meditation increases tolerance of pain.
- Cardiovascular problems then cause greater anxiety, depression, and anger. Long-term stress and anxiety can be a vicious circle for the heart. Meditation breaks habitual patterns, releasing emotional factors.

In *Emotional Intelligence*, Daniel Goleman describes the following dangers of chronic anger:

- faster heart rate and higher blood pressure over the years
- resulting in a buildup of plaque in the arteries, causing coronary heart disease and blood clotting
- leading to myocardial infarction (heart attack) and stroke[109]

In this age of high anxiety and stress, he says, "...chronic hostility and repeated episodes of anger seem to put men at greatest risk for heart disease."[110]

Goleman goes on to suggest that depression may be another major emotional cause of heart disease:

> Noting that depression increases fivefold the likelihood of coronary heart disease, that kind of patient is at high risk. It's unethical to not start trying to treat these factors.[111]

As noted above, meditation is a known treatment for depression.

Thus, evidence for meditation as an indicated intervention in both the prevention and treatment of heart disease is well established.

Anxiety Care

Meditation is a widely known reducer of anxiety and stress. Benson said that people who meditate recover from stressful impacts faster, and they have fewer chronic or inappropriate emergency responses.[112] Calm presence of mind in people who practice meditation brings appropriate behavior to the circumstance.

Pelletier has observed that meditation is effective because it inhibits the negative patterns established in the sympathetic nervous system. Meditation breaks the patterns of incessant sympathetic arousal that are a correlate of anxiety states and are implicated in a range of stress related disorders ranging from hypertension to cancer.[113]

In the survey of the research literature on the effects of meditation cited in Murphy and Donovan's book, we find substantial evidence that meditation lowers heart rate, lowers blood pressure in people who are normal to moderately hypertensive, and normalizes irregularities of heart rhythm.[114] With respect to blood flow, they conclude:

> Meditation often helps relax the large muscle groups pressing on the circulatory system in various parts of the body. It might also relax the small muscles that control the vessels themselves; when that happens, the resulting elasticity of blood vessel walls would help reduce the pressure inside them.[115] ...
>
> The heart rates of both experienced and inexperienced meditators recovered from stressor impacts more quickly than control subjects, demonstrating a psychophysical configuration in stress situations opposite to that seen in stress-related syndromes... Meditation generally produces psychological results opposite from those of stress.[116]

Cancer Care

Though the causes of cancer may be less clear, there is some evidence that anxiety and fear may be significant factors, as they are well-known to impair immune function.

The extensive research at UMMC cited in this chapter has clearly established meditation as a proven method of reducing anxiety and stress and empowering immune system function. These results suggest that meditation can play a significant role in the treatment of cancer, in addition to any surgical, chemical, or radiation treatment employed.

Magarey[117] stated that medical technology has not reduced the death rate from cancer for 50 years, suggesting that a broader, more holistic approach, involving meditation is indicated. He pointed out that meditation is associated with physiological rest and stability, and also with the reduction of psychological stress and the development of a more positive attitude toward life, with an inner sense of calm, strength and fulfillment.[118]

In the more than thirty years since Magarey published the above statements concerning cancer, the death rate from cancer is relatively unchanged, but there has been an increase of the use of meditation in cancer therapy and there is now a better understanding of why it is indicated in cancer care. Murphy and Donovan cite a number of studies, including the following:

> Meares proposed a form of intensive meditation associated with the regression of cancer (1983); discussed the relationship between stress, meditation, and cancer (1982a, 1982b); reported on a case of regression of recurrence of carcinoma of the breast at a mastectomy site associated with intensive meditation (1981); reported the results of treatment of seventy- three patients with advanced cancer who attended at least twenty sessions of meditation and experienced significant reductions of anxiety and depression (1980a); reported on a case of remission of massive metastasis from undifferentiated carcinoma of the lung associated with intensive meditation (1980b); analyzed meditation as a psychological approach to cancer treatment (1979b); reported on a case of regression of cancer of the rectum after intensive meditation (1979a); analyzed the quality of meditation effective in the regression of cancer (1978a); reported on the regression of osteogenic sarcoma metastases associated with intensive meditation (1978c); looked at the relationship between vivid visualization and dim visual awareness in the regression of cancer after meditation (1978a); raised the issue of atavistic regression, which reportedly occurs in meditation, as a factor in the remission of cancer (1977); and reported on the case of a woman whose breast cancer was alleviated through intensive meditation (1976a). [119]

They also report on the case of a 43-year-old patient who used meditation as a treatment of last resort for diplopia and ataxia. Although the reason for the improvement his patient experienced in these diseases is elusive, Gersten believed that meditation was a significant factor in the healing process.[120]

Most importantly, in understanding the potential of mind-body medicine, we see that our potential for control over our somatic systems is greater than had been previously understood. Like biofeedback, the meditation experience can demonstrate to patients that they are capable of producing a shift in the body's functioning—

a profound change in their relationship to their body. Seeing that they have a measure of control over function can be both exhilarating and therapeutic. "Functions thought to be beyond conscious control were quite controllable with specialized practice."[121]

Meditation methods are biologically beneficial both because they give us a sense of control over biological process and, at the same time, because they give us detachment from the processes of mind that often impair our physiological function.

> ...reaching a detached state of mind for even 5 minutes a day is so valuable that it can infuse your body with the equivalent energy of 6 months of living in hope. [It's] a way of separating yourself from the fears of mind and viewing your circumstance as an experience through which you are passing rather than one that controls your physical life.[122]

Diabetes Care

Diabetes is another major cause of death in the West. It is an increasing health problem in developing countries, as well, where populations are shifting from traditional, vegetable and whole-grain oriented diets to the commercial Western diet, based on sugars, fats, salts, and starches. Such a diet exacts a toll on the pancreas, leading to insulin imbalances and ultimately the symptoms of diabetes.

Because blood flow and oxygenation are affected by meditation, and stress-related insulin secretions are reduced in the meditative states, positive results have been observed: Blood sugar levels of subjects with Type-2 diabetes practicing a meditation-relaxation technique were significantly reduced after participating in a 6-week program, whereas the blood sugar levels of subjects in a diabetes education program and a control group did not significantly change.[123]

Hospital Care

> In order to reduce fatalities and extended debility from surgery and overmedication, hospitals have increasingly been introducing meditation programs for surgery patients. Every surgeon knows that people who are extremely scared do terribly in surgery. They bleed too much; they have more infections and complications. They have a harder time recovering. It's much

Meditation Research

better if they are calm... Panic and anxiety hike blood pressure and veins distended by blood pressure bleed more profusely when cut by the surgeon's knife. Excess bleeding is one of the most troublesome complications and can lead to death.[124]

With respect to adverse drug reactions, it's been demonstrated that meditation is a remarkable pain management therapy; practitioners of meditation require less or no pain medication, thereby reducing drug intake that may be a factor.[125]

A New Medical Approach

We've written this book because we've seen that historical events have made a new kind of therapeutic method available to the world, and that access to knowledge of those methods is a basic right for all beings. As Deepak Chopra has said,

Knowledge can heal, and according to mind-body science, knowledge is the greatest healer of all.

The words medicine and meditation come from the same root, the Latin word *mediere*, meaning "to cure," and meditation has always had a close alignment with healing.

Medicine cures by eliminating the symptoms of a disorder. Meditation goes deeper, restoring physical and emotional balance and harmony through "right inward measure," which is one definition of healing. In short:

Medicine = curing the results of a condition;

Meditation = taking out the basis of a condition.

The research described in this chapter indicates that meditation methods have emerged as one of the "new" (though ancient) therapeutic methods, affecting many health conditions and offering people a way to live well with the challenges of our age. Meditation methods can enhance our ability to deal with this culture of Anxiety and reduce or eliminate a variety of health disorders.

Meditation is self-care, a self-applied skill, a unique medical art that can directly benefit health with no medical risk. Sitting to meditate, to relax and let the breath slow down and deepen, can be used as a complement to any allopathic medical treatment. In some cases it may be a complete medical path in itself, avoiding the risks of invasive medicine and enhancing patients' ability to improve their own physical and emotional function.

We've shared here that in the past 35 years more than 50,000 research papers and books have been published on the effectiveness of mind-body interventions in healthcare, with thousands of those demonstrating the effectiveness of meditation in reducing or eliminating a broad range of symptoms.

And, as the research continues to demonstrate, meditation, like all healing practices, does require faith in the method to use it well. Fortunately, the practice of meditation itself instills faith in its potential through its immediate effects. Most importantly, the practice of meditation restores faith in oneself as capable of self care, which becomes a great resource in the emerging era of healthcare.

಄

PART TWO: A NEW MODEL OF HEALING

The idea of a unified mind-body system as a basis for medical treatment is by no means established within Western scientific and medical circles—we are too early in the unfolding of this particular scientific revolution. It is, however, growing, and is founded in a long history of experience and recent clinical experiments. Taken together, these suggest and call for a new model of the human being, one that explains these research results and offers new possibilities for medical treatment.

States of Consciousness—Emerging Understandings

During the 1960s and '70s, while meditation was being introduced to the US, college students and faculty were engaged in explorations into the effects of various chemicals and were recording results that remarkably paralleled the descriptions shared by mystics across religious traditions down through the centuries. As the results of all this exploration and research filtered through the psychology research community, fascinating questions were raised—questions that challenged basic assumptions about the nature of mind and consciousness.

Two opposing schools of psychology emerged out of the process. One was the structuralist-materialists, for whom all awareness, consciousness, thought, and emotions were a product of the chemical interactions of the brain. The other was the transpersonalists, for whom personal consciousness was the dynamic result of the interaction of cultural, physiological, and other processes going on within and around the individual, not always definable.

A significant contributor to the dialogue between these groups was a meticulous experimental psychologist at the University of California, Davis, Charles T. Tart, Ph.D.. He felt compelled to respond to the phenomena going on around him. As he described it:

> In the last month two graduate students in physics have come to talk to me about their experiences of their "souls leaving their bodies"; a sociology graduate student told me about a group of students he meets with regularly to discuss what to do with your state of consciousness and style of life after exhausting the LSD-25 experience; a mathematics graduate student asked for a guide to the scientific literature on marijuana . . .[126]

Unable to address these questions in traditional psychological terms, Tart set out to develop an experimental framework and language for identifying, describing, and predicting the processes associated with the growing body of experiential evidence.

In his early book, *Altered States of Consciousness*, Tart collected some of the most precise descriptions of experiences available in the literature, exploring the nature of dream consciousness, hypnagogic states, hypnosis, and states induced by the use of psychedelic drugs. In the introduction to this collection, he states:

> An altered state of consciousness [ASC] for a given individual is one in which he clearly feels a qualitative shift in his pattern of mental functioning, that is, he feels not just a quantitative shift (more or less alert, more or less visual imagery), but also that some quality or qualities of his mental processes are different. [127]

According to Tart, every culture has its own attitudes toward ASCs. Some respect ASCs for potential wisdom, and some fear them. Mind has changed throughout history and attitudes toward ASCs change. In America today, the fields of psychology and psychiatry have shown insufficient interest in altered states.

In a later volume, entitled simply *States of Consciousness*, Tart applies a systems approach to the material he had accumulated over nearly a decade of research. In the process, he develops a model of the various states of consciousness that every individual moves through in the course of a day, or a lifetime and comes to a new way of thinking about consciousness. He distinguishes between awareness and consciousness, saying that awareness is knowledge that something is happening, elemental perceiving or feeling. Consciousness, he says, is more complex. It's modulated by the mind:

> I would use the word awareness to describe, for instance, my simple perception of the sound of a bird... I would use the word consciousness to indicate the complex of operations that recognizes a sound as a bird call, that identifies the species of bird.[128]

As Tart continued to work with both the language and the experiences he was encountering, he developed a model that differs significantly from the familiar "conservative" understanding of mind as the product of sensory input and chemical interaction. Tart's model describes consciousness as a complex process of distinguishing and relating that is shaped by one's cultural, familial, educational, and experiential background. In his model, consciousness is informed by "pure awareness," which is "something that comes from outside the structure of the physical brain, as well as something influenced by the structure of the brain."[129]

This idea of pure awareness as coming from outside the brain is, he says,

> "...a most unpopular idea in scientific circles, but... there is enough scientific evidence that consciousness is capable of temporarily existing in a way that seems independent of the physical body..."[130]

Later he distinguished between "awareness" and "attention," saying that the latter is "how we direct" awareness.

A second aspect of Tart's model that was "unpopular in scientific circles" is the idea that "physical reality is not a completely fixed entity, but something that may actually be shaped in some fundamental manner by the individual's beliefs about it."[131] As an example, he refers to an experience described by Joseph Chilton Pearce in *The Crack in the Cosmic Egg* in which Pearce was temporarily convinced he was impervious to pain and "ground out the tips of glowing cigarettes on his cheeks, palms, and eyelids . . . felt no pain, and there was no sign of physical injury."[132] Tart points out that, in material terms, the tip of a cigarette has such a high temperature that it must burn the skin—yet the skin was not burned; hence physical reality was shaped in some way by Pearce's temporary, hypnosis-induced belief.

The third major contribution of Tart's model of states of consciousness is the understanding that what we call "ordinary consciousness" is not a particular discrete state. What is "normal" or "ordinary" varies from culture to culture, from individual to individual, and from situation to situation. For example, the state of consciousness in which we drive a car or watch television is very different from that in which we cook a meal or repair a bicycle—they are waking states but use very different modes of functioning, show very different brain-wave patterns, and light up different areas of the brain on scanners.

As a result, Tart discarded the language of "Altered States" of consciousness and replaced it with "Discrete States," suggesting that we experience a continuum of states of consciousness over the course of the day, each of which has its own distinguishing characteristics.

In this, Tart's work supports and reflects that of the great pioneer of psychology, William James, who said in a paper published in 1898:

Our normal waking consciousness is but one special type of consciousness, while all about it, parted from it by the filmiest of screens, there lie potential forms of consciousness entirely different. We may go through life without suspecting their existence, but apply the requisite stimulus and at a touch they are there in all their completeness.[133]

A Continuum

If we consider our experience over the course of a day, we can begin to understand the various states of consciousness we move through. Immediately prior to awaking we are usually dreaming, a state of consciousness that involves particular brain functions and has its own "laws" of operation. As we move into our day, we may sit with a beverage and become engrossed in a news story in the paper or on television—we've entered a new state of consciousness in which alpha waves dominate the brain function and the sensory system filters out unrelated external inputs. We shower, dress, and move out into the world in the "ordinary" consciousness of activity—unless we happen to have been daydreaming in the process. On the bus or train, or in the elevator, fragments and sets of thoughts shift constantly through undefined states and we are once more all but oblivious to external events, until we are startled out of our reverie—into another state of consciousness—by our arrival at our destination. And so forth.

Even without the use of medications, drugs, or mind-altering methods, we have already experienced several states of consciousness and we haven't even begun the day's work!

States of consciousness, then, are best understood not as "normal" and "altered," but as a continuum of cognitive functions.

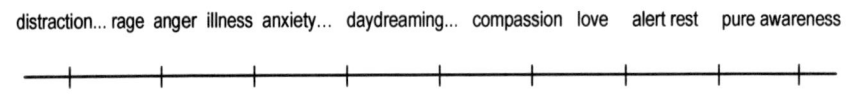

distraction... rage anger illness anxiety... daydreaming... compassion love   alert rest   pure awareness
—+————+————+————+————+————+————+————+————+—

A continuum of states of consciousness.

Near the center of that continuum might be the states associated with conversation, completing familiar tasks, or exploring something new and interesting. At one extreme, we can place the state in which we experience pure awareness—undistracted awareness without limit, free of the obstruction created by thought and emotion. At the other end is total distraction—that is, continual responding to every external stimulus with both emotions and evaluative processes. States such as those associated with "the zone" in sports and creativity, or with the creative movement of dancing, would come between daydreaming and "alert rest." The states in which we experience overwhelm, anger, and upset can be placed closer to the "total distraction" extreme.

Other Western Models

If we look at the history of psychology, we see that many great thinkers have explored the nature of consciousness and mind, with some very effective models. Most of those developed in the nineteenth and twentieth centuries were attempts to explain behavioral pathologies and abnormalities. Freud's famous "ego, superego, id" model is perhaps the best known of these, but his students Carl Jung and Roberto Assagioli each developed models that sought to explain the different forms of human function and the therapeutic interventions that fit their experience. Jung's tends to be transpersonal in nature, relating the individual consciousness to a shared human, or collective, consciousness, while Assagioli's, though far more complex, tends to remain within the structural-physical realm of the individual.

All of these models are useful in understanding the processes by which pathologies and other undesirable patterns develop and can be treated. None of them, however, were designed to explain the different states of conscious-ness that each of us experience on a moment-to-moment basis.

Another approach to consciousness was the cybernetic model of mind functioning offered by neurologist H. Ross Ashby, who used the language of cybernetics to synthesize what became the basis for a "bio-computer" model of the brain-mind system.[134] At the other extreme, Gregory Bateson took some of the same cybernetic concepts to develop "an ecology of mind," in which mental process was seen as a function of the interacting totality of the individual as part of family, workplace, culture, and ecosystem.[135]

Outside the realm of theoretical or clinical psychology, however, another set of models has been emerging. One model that was developed in the early twentieth century begins to explore the nature of consciousness for its own sake. Georges Gurdjieff, born in Armenia and trained in various Eastern traditions, taught a number of Sufi-based consciousness-altering techniques. He stated it in terms of identity states:

"Every thought, every mood, every desire, every sensation, says 'I'... Man's every thought and desire appears and lives quite separately and independently of the Whole. And the Whole never expresses itself... Man is divided into a multiplicity of small I's." [136]

Gurdjieff's recommendation for understanding these various "I"s, or moments of being, was self-observation, and he provided a wide range of tools for his students to use in that process. One of his students, P. D. Ouspensky, expanded on his teachings and methods through the 1940s and '50s, linking them to 20th-century psychological models in his best known book, *In Search of the Miraculous*.

Students of esoteric psychology have developed a number of models to explain both the formation of patterns of mind functioning and the experiences that Tart has defined as "Discrete States of Consciousness." Of these, perhaps the most widely read is Alice Bailey.

In *From Intellect to Intuition*, Bailey identified five stages, or states, of consciousness to be achieved through the practice of *raja yoga* as she understood it. These are:

1. concentration,
2. meditation,
3. contemplation,
4. illumination, and
5. inspiration.

Each of these states builds on the last, with meditation made possible by the experience of concentration, the depth of contemplation enabled by the experience of meditation, and so on. As did Gurdjieff, Bailey found that the path through these states is self-observation—both in stillness and in action.

States of Consciousness—Emerging Understandings   83

    Two classics from the 1970s are Robert Ornstein's *Psychology of Consciousness* and Charles Hampden-Turner's *Maps of the Mind*. They provide compilations of the many theories and models of mental functions that enable the reader to place these ideas into some framework of distinctions and similarities. Neither of them, however, provide a framework for working with the specific states of consciousness that we typically experience—and the others that we have the capacity to experience—in the course of our lives.

    A wonderful exploration of consciousness observed is Itzhak Bentov's *Stalking the Wild Pendulum*. Integrating the "hard sciences" of physics and chemistry with the "soft sciences" of psychology and anthropology, Bentov suggests that normal, waking consciousness is a small part of our total consciousness, pointing out that "in an altered state of consciousness we can expand our subjective time greatly."[137] This corresponds with the findings of Robert Masters and Jean Houston, who provided guidelines for what they call "accelerated mental processes" in their classic handbook for guided visualization, *Mind Games*.

    Bentov goes on to define a "state of being" as experiencing the totality of consciousness, or "the absolute." He suggests that meditation practices help us to achieve that "state of being", that in that state we integrate the various aspects and states of consciousness that we've experienced over our lives and also begin to sense the information and intelligence of other consciousnesses.[138]

Depth of States and Opportunities for Development

    As Tart continued to work with the states of consciousness reported in the literature and by his experimental subjects, he came to understand that within each state resided a range of potential experience. He noted that this range was not made up of distinctly different qualities, or states, of consciousness—but was, rather, a matter of more or less of the same qualities. He called this potential for more or less, "depth."[139]

    Tart observed that as one goes deeper into a state of consciousness, the intensity of the qualities of that state tends to increase, until at a certain point—which varies by state—the intensity remains constant, while the depth may continue to increase. For example, one may be reading and reach a point where the internally generated images are clear and crisp while still being aware at some level of one's environment, and gradually become less and less aware of anything but the images associated with one's reading, although they are no clearer than before.

Tart's research suggests that consciousness may be experienced in any one of many states, with greater or lesser depth or intensity in each state. We may develop our capacity to enter into different states at will, and to increase or decrease the depth and intensity of our experience in each state. Then, as we learn to experience increased depth in a particular state of consciousness, we experience increased ability to maintain that state and to prolong its effects on the mind-body system.

Thus deep anxiety can lead to illness, while deep meditation can lead to improved mind-body functioning well after the meditation period is completed.

Eastern Models

The nature of consciousness has been the core study of Buddhist and Hindu yogis for more than two thousand years, and a very refined working knowledge of the cognitive potential evolved through the research, teachings, and literature of those traditions. Some of that literature was made available, in translation, as early as the mid-1800s, but it's only since the Tibetan diaspora that Westerners have had the opportunity to really study and comprehend the depth of the Buddhist model. By now hundreds of books have been published in English to help facilitate the transfer of information.

Yoga

The ancient Sanskrit *Vedas* (5,000 to 8,000 years old) provide the basis for much of the Hindu and Buddhist model, expanded by the *Upanishads* (about a thousand years old) and codified in the *Yoga Sutras* of Patanjali, who is variously reported to have written anywhere from 600 to 1,600 years ago.

A number of translations of Patanjali's *Sutras* are available and a number of Hindu yogis have written English texts to help us to understand the variations on the Hindu model. Perhaps the most famous of these is by Christopher Isherwood and Swami Prabhavananda, entitled *How to Know God,* which is oriented toward

States of Consciousness—Emerging Understandings 85

the Vedanta school. Many later translations are available, but we will rely on Archibald Bahm's *Yoga Sutras of Patanjali* for his simple and clear overview of the model.

Each of the several hundred Sutras is a statement that provides the basis for an interpretive reading or lecture. Patanjali's statements are the introductions to a series of lectures on the nature and practice of something that was referred to often in the ancient texts but never fully explained—hence the popularity of his work.

The practices of yoga are designed to free the self from any mental disturbance that might prevent union with the ultimate reality. These disturbances may be enjoyable or distressing, but all prevent the desired union.

Patanjali defines two kinds of consciousness, which is consistent with the Buddhist model we will explore next.. Bahm translates those as "normal consciousness... occupied with investigating, distinguishing, enjoyment, and selfconsciousness" and "superior consciousness" that "has freed itself from such occupation."

He says that everyone may attain "superior consciousness" and that several factors contribute to the ease of that attainment, including one's natural tendencies, one's faith and commitment, and one's "wholehearted emulation of the Ideal Soul."("Ideal Soul" is Bahm's translation of the Sanskrit word *Ishwara*, which is often translated as "God.") He points out that Patanjali's next sutras define the Ishwara in terms that are not consistent with the Western idea of God:

> The Ideal Soul serves as the Supreme Example... being timeless it exists at all times... the traditional symbol 'OM' applies to it.[136]

Patanjali's next sutra recommends repetition of the sound "OM," with comprehension of its significance, as an aid in progressing toward superior consciousness—and Bahm reminds us that this form of repetition

> involves a giving of one's whole self to domination by attention to intonation of the universal, omnisonorous, self-contained meaning which it embodies. [137]

This is another method for the return to primal health.

As the sutras progress, Patanjali explains the various obstructions of normal consciousness and describes the various pitfalls one may encounter along the way. Then he begins to describe the experience of "superior conciousness".

When one enjoys consciousness entirely freed from desire for results, then the true nature of all things becomes clear.[138]

Through the several hundred sutras, Patanjali explains how the mind and body are enhanced with the practice. In the final sutra we are told, "the soul, as pure awareness, remains perfectly pure".[139] It's the key to the health of body, mind, and spirit. Inherent free awareness is the key to unconditioned life.

Another yoga tradition, called *Kriya* (from the roots *kri*, "action," and *ya*, "awareness") *Yoga*, was brought to the West by Paramahansa Yogananda and is now offered in the Self-Realization Fellowship. This form teaches that there are four states of consciousness:

1. physical consciousness: present during daily activities

2. dream consciousness: present during astral

experiences or in waking mental activities

3. consciousness during deep sleep without dreams

4. pure consciousness: "turiya," . . . beyond the

three others, their source, eternal, infinite without

modification.[140]

Although this tradition is closely related to, and draws somewhat upon, the teachings of Patanjali, the focus is on the methods taught by Kriya Babaji Nagaraj as presented by Yogiar Ramaiah in Tamil Nadu, India, and clarified by Yogananda's teacher, Ishtewar. These involve postures, movements, and visualization, as well as breath control. The ultimate goal of *kriya yoga* is to achieve a state of consciousness that is so much in union with the ultimate, so consistently turiya, that the body is transformed into the "Effulgence of God" and disappears into light.[141]

Tibetan Buddhist

Though there are four lineages of Tibetan Buddhist teaching, each with its own nuances, they share fundamental principles. *The Tibetan Book of Living and Dying* by Sogyal and the books of Chogyam Trungpa are particularly useful in helping us understand these fundamentals.

States of Consciousness—Emerging Understandings

In the Tibetan Buddhist model, as in the Hindu yoga model, there are two principles of human experience:

- *rigpa*— "pure awareness," free of any tendency, "the radiant ground of all existence," unmoving, primordial wisdom;
- *alaya*— "storehouse consciousness," the potential to create all effects of karma, the tendency of mind to create life and death, and the tendency to develop multiple kinds of consciousness.

The Tibetan word *rigpa* is in Sanskrit *vidya*, which comes from root meanings "to know, to understand, perceive," and "to act". Thus it can denote the action of knowing or understanding, with some emphasis on perceiving or seeing an object. And at some levels of the meditative process, such "knowing" is indeed experienced.

But at its deepest level there is no longer any separation between the seeing and the seen, the knowing and the known, between the meditator and the object of meditation. In the deepest state achieved through meditation one is resting in *rigpa*, free awareness, and not reacting to the eight consciousnesses, or kinds of tendency, thus breaking the unstable dynamic of form and action, the pattern we call *karma*. In *rigpa* we return, in unmoving awareness, to the stable basis of health, the basis of psychological sanity, psychological health, and physiological homeostasis.

Although some traditions see the *alaya* consciousness as the void from which all form emerges, practitioners in the Nyingma lineage of Buddhist teachings see *rigpa* as what is also called *Dharmakaya*, a state of pure awareness that is free of *alaya* and the other 7 forms of consciousness. As the potential of everything, the *Dharmakaya* is the space from which *alaya* and the other 7 consciousnesses emerge.

In this understanding the 8 kinds of consciousness are usually listed as follows:

#1–5 are the five sense consciousnesses (seeing, smelling, hearing, tasting, and touching), understood as forms of projection;

#6, the "mind," which uses the five senses;

#7 can be called the subconscious tendencies of mind;

#8 is the *alaya*, which breaks into the above tendencies dynamically through its creative energy. (*Alaya* is Sanskrit; in Tibetan the word is *kunzhi* and means "the foundation of all things." It's the ground of all materiality, where karmic, or cause/effect, imprints are stored. It's the source of what Taoists call "the ten thousand things," or the material universe.)

These eight consciousnesses are the eight ways we project our beliefs and expectations onto the otherwise empty or formless void. We project them many times each minute through the sense consciousnesses, through the "conscious mind," and through the unconscious and subconscious tendencies. This tendency is called *dzinpa* in Tibetan.

These projections are how we experience form, and then we react to the forms we project as if they were "out there" "coming at us" rather than projections of our own mental state.[140] This process creates further tendencies in us to react in similar ways, which is called *karma*.

However, the state of being called *rigpa*, awareness itself or "the radiant ground of all existence," is free of the limitations of form or feeling and the key to unconditioned life. Our experience of *rigpa* is open, spacious, and expansive in nature. Free of form and unaffected by *karma*, free of *alaya* and the other 7 consciousnesses, the experience of *rigpa* is the inherent key to health and a new healthcare system.

Meditation Methods & States of Consciousness

While awareness is open and free of self-preoccupation, mind is constantly talking and thinking about itself. Mind is best understood as the constantly changing, self-centered, conceptual activity of our normal thought processes, intensely concerned with time. Mind is most often not even really focused on the present, tending to be involved with past and future. This means that the practice of intentional return to unconditioned awareness is a healthful release of unhealthy tendencies.

Mind & Awareness

At the moment of the shift from mind to awareness, mind attaches to that shift and is proud of itself, claiming to have made the shift. In the process, it becomes attached to the activity of meditation in accordance with its *dzinpa* tendency.

Awareness recognizes this tendency of mind, and is inherently free of it. This is because both mind and the shift back to awareness are discontinuous and awareness is continuous. It has an unmoving, unchanging quality. Awareness is unaffected by the practice of meditation.

Awareness is always present; it's what people come home to when they shift attention out of the trances of mind back into living presence, where life is. Awareness is inborn, inherently free of mind. Awareness is a free, unconditioned alternative to our normal, conditioned mind.

In distinguishing between mind and awareness it helps to recognize two aspects of mind: grasping and fixation. Mind is developed through these two interacting tendencies of grasping (attachment to objects) and fixation (attachment to self) Grasping is outwardly directed, attachment to the apparent phenomena of the world, defining the world in terms of one's own limited story. Fixation is inwardly directed attachment to the apparent subject of experience: "I," "me."

Through the process of observing our thoughts, we see that we fixate on ourselves because mind is afraid of losing what it calls itself, the subject of experience, which is sometimes called "ego" or "small self." The interactions of these tendencies form our thought processes and actions, which in turn limit and obstruct our capacity to be aware.

In his exploration into the nature of consciousness, Bentov suggests:

> ...we can equate the state of being with the absolute, since both imply no motion, no action, and total rest. At the same time, though, it is a state of high potential energy, because this state of rest is infinitely fast motion... tremendous energy and full of creative potential... plus intelligence. This intelligence adds a self-organizing capability.[141]

Awareness is effortless, the basis for healing release. Thus, in *rigpa*, the experiences of psychological freedom, physical wellbeing, and panoramic awareness are inseparable. Unlike the mind with its constant effort to maintain its projections, pure awareness requires no effort to achieve or to sustain, and so the mind-body system can allow a balanced energy flow to and through the cells and organs.

Pure awareness has the potential to enable the body to heal and evolve. This is why all the research into the mind-body functioning of meditators shows high levels of functioning across the mind-body system. As we saw in Chapter Three, people who meditate regularly—almost regardless of meditation method—have better-than-average blood pressure, heart rate, hormone balances, immune function, muscle tone, cerebral functioning, recall, and comprehension. Pure awareness has no form or action, so the mind-body system can rest from response and reaction, allowing its creative processes to resume and restore the body.

Meditation as a Means, Not a State

When meditation methods were first introduced to Westerners there was a widely held belief that meditation itself was a particular state of consciousness. Bailey presented it as such in her stages, and even Tart described it as such in his early work on "Altered States".[142] Although the ultimate goal of the meditation process may be to experience the unified state of being that Buddhists call *rigpa* and Hindus call *turiya* or *nirvana*, (the experience of which is called *Samadhi*) and the Abramic traditions (including Islam, Judaism, and Christianity) call ecstatic Union with God,[143] not all meditation methods are designed to achieve that end.

As Tart discovered, and as research on the variety of Eastern meditation experiences continued, it became clear that meditation is not a unique state, but a means by which the individual can experience various levels of depth or intensity in any one of several states of consciousness—all of which may be located on the continuum of states illustrated earlier in this chapter.

If we consider the many meditation methods available to us today, we can see that a range of depths, intensities, and states may be achieved. Some methods, like progressive neuromuscular release, shift our attention in a way that calms the mind-body system. Some, like focusing on a mantra or flame or flower, discipline the mind to concentrate and may begin to dissolve perceived boundaries between self and other. Some, like guided visualization or shamanic journeys, lead to an expanded perception of time, space, and the nature of reality. And so forth.

All of these methods accomplish two things: they stop the habitual thought process and they restore a measure of harmony and balance in the mind-body system so that its interacting patterns of thoughts, emotions, and physiological processes are mutually supportive, no longer dysfunctional. In short, they encourage healing.

New Understandings of the Body

The scientific advances of the 20th and early 21st centuries have gone well beyond the model of human anatomy and function that is the basis for what Dr. Larry Dossey has called Era I, scientific-reductionist medicine. As we discussed earlier in this book, a number of Era II mind-body therapies have been demonstrated as effective healing methods within the Western scientific paradigm, and are now collectively referred to as "complementary and alternative medicine" or CAM.

These methods use different healing modalities and point to new understandings about the nature of the body and mind. So, since an appropriate vision of the human body and mind is essential for understanding and applying the methods associated with the new expanded medical treatment, we will try to present such an integrated model here.

As we've come to understand it, an integrated model of the dynamic, multi-dimensional human being appropriate for an expanded paradigm of medical science would have to:

- describe a body that is dynamically responsive at every level of function.
- explain the effectiveness of mental and physical therapies working outside the scientific-reductionist paradigm of Western medicine;
- describe a role for the range of interacting electromagnetic fields that are continually being measured in and around in the body;
- explain the presence of and the effectiveness of therapies manipulating energy within the body (called variously, universal life energy, *chi*, *prana*, life force, or the fifth force);

Contributions to such a model must necessarily come from many disciplines, and from ancient, as well as contemporary scientists. To this end, we've drawn on the work of many researchers, from both contemporary and historically significant traditions. Biochemists, medical practitioners, and systems theorists, cellular and molecular biologists, quantum theorists and biophycisits, and yogis, as well as cyberneticians and metaphysicians, all inform our model.

The Energetic Mind-Body

A new set of understandings about the nature of matter and the human mind-body emerged in the 20th century sciences, which must necessarily change our way of thinking about the mind and body.

Living Systems

Through the last decades of the 20th century, as mathematicians, ecologists, and systems thinkers explored the behavior and evolution of complex systems, the set of ideas called Living Systems Theory emerged. It integrates these disciplines into a body of principles that apply to all living organisms and social organizations.

The first principle of all systems theory is that everything is interconnected so we can never do just one thing. In a simple machine, it's possible to remove one part and insert another, similar one without affecting much in the system's functioning. As the machine becomes more complex, however, such removal and replacement can have unexpected consequences. And when internal governance, such as a thermostat, is part of the machine, it becomes a system, and no part can be changed without changing the way the whole system functions. (You cannot, for example, put the fuel injectors of a sports car into a mini-van or diesel truck.)

In living systems, this is even more the case: one cannot affect a part of a body without affecting many other parts of the body. One cannot, for example, injure a foot without affecting the joints of the leg and the overall posture, which may lead to spinal injury at the worst—or simply an aching back and shoulders as the muscles do unaccustomed work. Nor can we introduce a chemical—say, an antibiotic to kill an infectious bacterium—without affecting other aspects of the system; the antibiotic will also kill the "good" bacteria that live in the intestines and help us digest foods. Similarly, the use of a pain-killer will affect the way the cells handle other proteins.

A second principle of Living Systems Theory is that even when things look chaotic, there is order; and vice versa: the most orderly processes include a degree of chaos. The underlying order of an apparently random forest or pond may not be evident until a part is injured or removed—then the resulting shifts and changes will demonstrate the order that was present, though not visible, before. Likewise, the orderly process of development from infant to adult seems, at times, to be chaotic, but in hindsight we can see how each individual event contributes to, and often contains the pattern of, the whole process.

A third principle of Living Systems Theory is nonlinearity. As Alan Watts, a British Anglican priest who traveled to Japan and became a well-known Buddhist philosopher, used to say, "Nature is wiggly." Living systems don't grow in a straight line; they grow exponentially, following an "S" shaped curve on a graph, and are sustainable within a range of limits between which they oscillate over time. Continuous growth is as unhealthy in living systems as is continuous decline—and will almost invariably lead to catastrophic results. A cycle of growth and decline, activity and rest, is the only sustainable pattern.

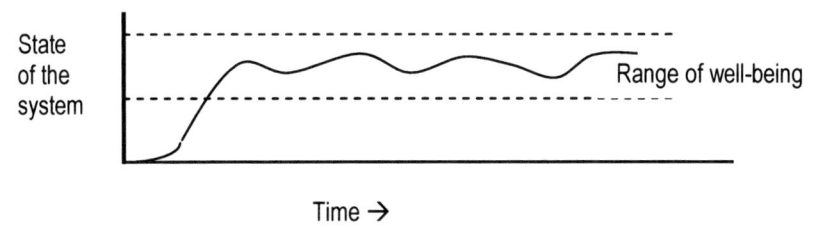

State of the system | Range of well-being

Time →

A fourth principle is that they are "dissipative structures." The term was coined by Nobel laureate Ilya Prigogine to describe the process by which many systems exist only as long as a consistent supply of energy continues to flow into them and through them. A whirlpool only exists as long as water flows through it at a near-constant flow rate. Similarly for tornadoes and electrical systems.

We can see how this works also with food in the body—too much, too fast, or not enough for long enough, and the body begins to malfunction. We can also see how it works with light and nourishment for plants. As long as energy continues to flow through the system within a certain range of intensity, the system is maintained. The effect of sunlight on the human body is less obvious, but as anyone who's dealt with Seasonal Affective Disorder because of lack of direct sunlight in the Pacific Northwest knows, a minimum flow of photons in certain energy ranges (associated with sunlight) is necessary for our wellbeing. At the same time, we all know that too much sunlight, or too much heat, or even too much food, is harmful to the body and can destroy the body system.

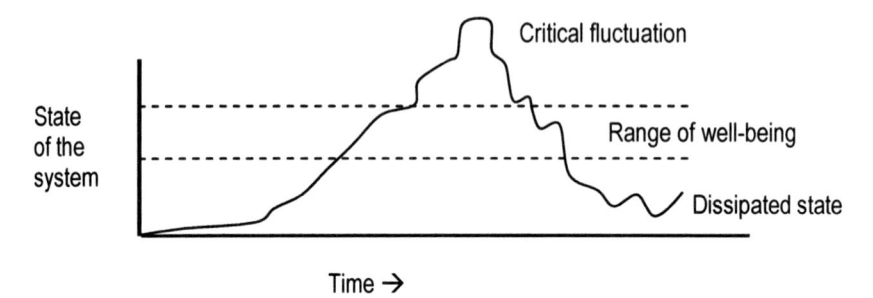

State of the system — Critical fluctuation — Range of well-being — Dissipated state — Time →

Several years after Prigogine's work was published, the "Iron Curtain" separating the Soviet Union from the rest of the world was dissolved (which process in itself is an illustration of Prigogine's theory) and the Western world saw the great distress that much of the Soviet Bloc had been living under. We were particularly saddened by the children in orphanages who, for lack of sufficient staff, had not been touched, hugged, or cuddled for most of their young lives. Parents who adopted those children have reported many psychological and some medical problems resulting from the lack of that particular form of energy, and have found that, for some of those children, social adaptation has been difficult and there's a propensity for certain diseases. This experience suggests that it's possible to describe "love" as a form of energy essential for the development and maintenance of the body as well as the person as a social being, along with the measurable energy in food and heat and light.

Prigogine also suggests that when the flow that sustains the structure changes suddenly or significantly, the structure may collapse or dissipate, or it may respond by restructuring in a way that can be

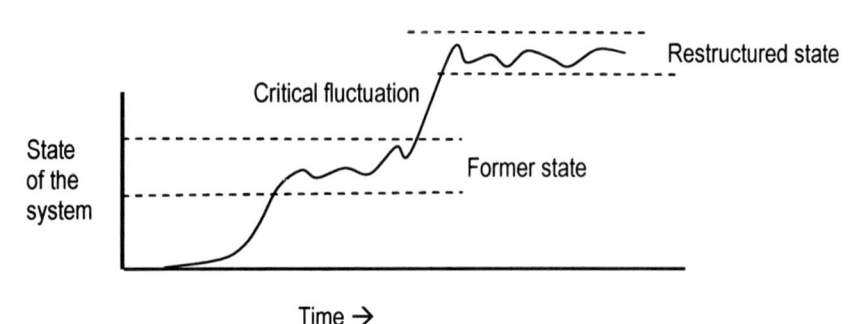

State of the system — Restructured state — Critical fluctuation — Former state — Time →

sustained with the new level of energy flow. Many researchers have used this principle to explain the evolutionary processes by which living systems increase in complexity.[144]

This increase in complexity happens through the fifth principle: living systems self-organize through the exchange of information in feedback mechanisms. All living systems develop from apparently inert "seeds of potentiality" into complex, dynamic bodies through the constant flow and exchange of information.

This means living systems are not subject to entropy. Unlike mechanical systems, which tend to wear down into dust, living systems are negentropic. Rather than simply decaying, life forms take in matter and energy from their environment, combine it in unique patterns, and form new structures with new capabilities through a series of developmental stages. Information about the environment, what's been taken in, the current state of being, and its outputs into the environment is transmitted throughout the system. This information is then "fed back" to the various processors in the system to adjust the level and direction of their activity and maximize life.

A living systems perspective, therefore, says that the human mind-body is:

> an interconnected whole within a larger interconnected whole, within which we can "never do just one thing." The mind-body constantly develops, in an orderly process that sometimes feels chaotic and is "wiggly" rather than linear. It's maintained by a continuous flow of energy and, if that flow shifts, the mind-body must restructure to function at the new level or it will dissipate or collapse into illness and, ultimately, death.

The flow of energy that sustains us, however, is not just the energy that's in our food or the light or heat or magnetism that can be measured on the electromagnetic spectrum. There is as yet no physical measure within Western science for the subtle energy we call Life; there's only the experience of it as the tendency of life forms to grow and develop: what some call "the negentropic factor."

Universal Energy Sustaining the Body

The Vedic (Hindu and Buddhist) traditions, however, offer rich explanations for this flow of energy. As Dharma Singh Khalsa, MD tells us,

> When you breathe, you don't just breathe in a gaseous mixture containing oxygen. You also breathe in prana, the universal life force. The ancient yoga masters were far more interested in the ethereal aspect of breathing than in the obvious physical aspect.[145]

What are the energies that can be breathed? The constantly flowing subtle energy that earned the Nobel Prize for biochemist Ilya Prigogine has long been called *prana* or *chi* in the Eastern meditation sciences. Eastern traditions call them the life-energy of the universe.

Traditionally this energy is differentiated into internal and external *chi* or *prana*. Most traditions describe both forms of life-energy, inner and universal, as the same "vital force," permeating all matter in different degrees.

The Vedic cultures of India and Tibet say *prana* is the vital force that is the difference between animate and inanimate objects. *Prana* is omnipresent and universal, the power generating life, a vital energy alive in the air. Meditation science says that *prana* can be experienced and breathed without being seen or felt.

The concept is not isolated to the Vedic cultures. The Greek word *pneuma* refers to both "spirit" and "breath" and the English word inspiration literally means "to breathe in." In Tibetan, the translation of *prana* is *lung*, which also means air or wind or psychic energy. The Japanese word for the universal energy, Ki, also means air. In Chinese, the fundamental universal energy field is called *chi*, the life force of the living body.

It's because of the natural affinity of the *prana* of the "external" universal/quantum field for the *prana* of the human body, in the "internal" quantum field, that *prana* is breathable. This fundamental, vital, subtle, information-energy is in the air, different from air and one with air at the same time. It can be sensed and breathed. According to a 19th century text by yoga master Ramacharaka,

> We are constantly inhaling the air charged with prana, and are as constantly extracting the latter from the air and appropriating it to our uses. Prana is found in its freest state in the atmospheric air, which when fresh is fairly charged with it, and we draw it to us more easily from the air than from any other source. In ordinary breathing we absorb and extract a normal supply of prana, but by controlled and regulated breathing (generally

known as Yogi breathing) we are enabled to extract a greater supply, which is stored away in the brain and nerve centers, to be used when necessary.[146]

In the *kriya yoga* tradition offered by Paramahansa Yogananda, *prana* is understood as the "nerve force" without which:

> the heart cannot beat, the lungs cannot breathe; the blood cannot circulate and the various organs cannot perform their respective normal functions. This prana not only supplies electric force to the nerves, but it also magnetizes the iron in the system and produces the aura as a natural emanation... the student of yogic breathing can actually feel the flow of energy throughout the network of nadis during each breath.[147]

Tibetan Vajrayana meditation practitioners learn to intentionally breathe, absorb, and optimize the function of, the *prana* or *lung* in the body. There it can be understood as having five qualities, much as light is seen to have five qualities. These qualities are called the "five airs", flowing in the subtle energy channels of the manifest body. These may be translated in terms of their form of operation, they are:

1. all-pervading in the body
2. circulating upward
3. circulating downward
4. preventing deterioration
5. holding life force

This understanding is a small fragment of a substantial body of mostly unpublished knowledge transmitted from teacher to student and is described more fully in the Appendix. It's taught as part of the processs of breathing the *prana* energy into the Life Vase (*Tse Bum*) in the lower abdomen (or womb), intentionally enhancing the functioning of the five *lungs* or *pranas* in the body. This form of breathing prana into the body is the basis for the method described in Part Three of this book as Awareness-based Energy Breathing.

What does Western science call lung/prana/chi? That these terms are now accepted by the National Institutes of Health suggests that Western scientific medicine has accepted the possibility of a distinct life energy. At the least, it's understood as the energy that Prigogine describes as essential for maintaining the integrity of any living system, whose flow literally maintains the structure and function of the mind-body.

In terms of modern physics, we could say that lung/prana/chi is not truly either energy or matter, but rather the flowing substrate of the quantum field, from which all matter and energy arise. This field may be experienced as the "clear light" of Buddhism or the "ground of being" of Hinduism. Amit Goswami, in his *The Self-Aware Universe* suggests that this field is consciousness itself.

It's the subtle energy from which all matter evolves, the creative energy of the void; it's the absolute potential from which the world of matter & energy emerges and which remains inseparable from the emergent matter. It can be described as "matter on the verge of becoming energy or energy on the point of becoming matter"[148] that is not yet measurable as energy and is sometimes referred to as the Universal Energy Field[149] or Zero-Point Field.[150] We'll explore more on this over the next few pages.

Semiconductors

Once we accept the possibility of various forms of energy as significant to the mind-body system, whole new possibilities emerge and we start to see relationships that have not been clear before.

Biologists studying the mechanism by which materials and information are passed through the outer "wall" or membrane of a cell, they have found two layers of permeable protein molecules with an impermeable layer of fat molecules between them ("like a butter sandwich," as Bruce Lipton says).

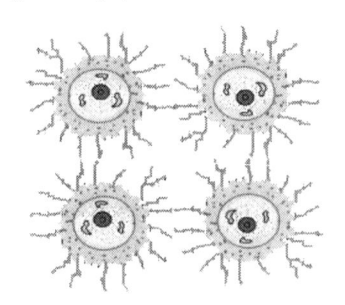

Not the nucleus, but the membrane, is the "brain" of the cell, and it's sensitive not just to chemical, but also electrical and subtler stimuli.

New Understandings of the Body

Through this, only the matter or information whose electrical charge pattern conforms to that of certain molecular gateways, called receptors, penetrates into the interior of the cell.

According to Lipton's *Biology of Belief*, this "semi-conducting" nature of the cell wall is part of how the cell maintains its identity in a constantly changing environment.[151]

Dr. Karl Maret has developed this vision further:

> ...medical schools and healers are not taught that the largest organ of the body is the connective tissue matrix. In the past this matrix was often simply seen as the stuff that glues the important organ systems of the body together. We are now realizing that it is here that the mysteries of life can be most fully explored...[152]

Maret challenges us further to shift our thinking about the body from a focus on the individual parts to the functioning whole.

> An inspired vision of this emerging medicine emphasizes the importance of the living tissue matrix with its... almost instantaneous, faster than nerve conduction, information transfer... Here cells are seen as fractals embedded in a holographic energetic matrix where everything is interconnected and capable of influencing every other part of the matrix. Information can be communicated through... photons of ultraviolet and visible light, phonons of sound, multiple resonant cellular vibrations, charge density waves and quantum potentials... Ultimately, a picture of an electro-magnetically unified matrix containing a self-organizing blueprint with innumerable feedback loops begins to emerge.[153]

Maret's vision helps us shift from a view of the mind-body limited by the solid structures we can measure with our usual senses to a tightly interconnected structure of electromagnetic processes that can only be measured with highly sensitive, high energy devices.

Liquid Crystals

The wave-form of our bodies is energy, but the matter-form of our bodies is mostly fluid. While an aged elder may have as little as 75% water making up the soft tissue, a child may have as much as 97%. Even the bones, when studied in the body, are soft and resilient—unlike the hard and dry skeletons that we are shown in museums and laboratories.

This fact is the fundamental basis for the turning point in the story-thread of the film *What the Bleep Do We Know?*. It's illustrated by the amazingly beautiful photographs of water crystals offered by Japanese researcher Mararu Emoto in his series of books, *Messages from Water*.

Emoto has established that the words, music, and even focused intention that surrounds a flask or pond of water can change that water's molecular structure. He demonstrates this by freezing water and observing it under the microscope as it changes from solid ice to frost. During the process the water forms different kinds of crystals—or none at all. Beautiful crystals result after thoughts and words of love, gratitude, and praise; none form with heavy-metal music, chemical treatments (i.e. tap water) or ugly words. This means, he says, that the water in our bodies and that we drink, swim, or fish in, is responding to what we're listening to, saying, and feeling—and may be helping our bodies or harming them as a result.[154]

The connective tissue of the material, or manifest body is, as we've said, mostly liquid. It takes the form of long, thin molecular structures that are known as "liquid crystals." These transmit and receive signals in the body just as they do in a cell phone, laptop, or flat screen TV. They make up a parallel system to the nerve system as part of the transfer of energy and information throughout the manifest body and it may be that this system is what generates the field that Maret and others have described—and distriburtes the lung/prana/chi.

Energy Body Channels

The subject of energy body anatomy has been of considerable public interest since the publication of *Hands of Light* by Barbara Brennan and *Anatomy of the Spirit* by Caroline Myss in the 1990s. As an explanation of the success of their methods, they offered a model that has been presented in the U.S. by teachers of various meditation science traditions since the 1970s and is based on some of the most ancient Hindu texts.

They describe a series of power centers, called *chakras*, aligned along a central energy channel that begins at the base of the spine and rises to above the head. Myss combines this model with other understandings of the body as a map for intuitive appreciation of

New Understandings of the Body

the energy dynamics of the individual. The *chakra* model comes from the ancient Sanskrit scientific texts, called the Vedas. In this understanding, the central energy channel, with its vertical series of seven to twelve *chakras* or energy centers, corresponds with the central nervous system and with glands of the endocrine system. For instance, the root chakra is traditionally located at the base of the spine and the crown chakra is traditionally associated with the cerebral cortex, while the "third eye" chakra is associated with the pineal gland and hypothalamus in the center of the brain.

This subtle or energy body model explains much of our internal experience and has provided the basis for many of the healing practices of Hindu and Buddhist cultures, some of which are offered in Part IV of this book. Here, we will be exploring the structure of that body as a way to understand why those methods work.

In *Vibrational Medicine,* Gerber states that there is

> ...considerable evidence to suggest that there exists a holographic energy template associated with the physical body... [within which] information is carried which guides the cellular growth of the physical structure of the body.... There are specific channels of energy exchange which allow the flow of energetic information to move from one system to another. [155]

Beyond their correspondence with aspects of the nervous and endocrine systems, the chakras, which may be pictured as dynamic energy wheels, are vortices of subtle energies. Gerber tells us they are:

> ...somehow involved in taking in higher [frequency] energies and transmuting them to a utilizable form within the human structure... From a physiologic standpoint, the chakras appear to be involved with the flow of higher energies via specific subtle energetic channels into the cellular structure of the human body. At one level they seem to function as transformers, stepping down energy of one form and frequency to a lower energetic level. [156]

This energy is transmuted through the systems of energy channels recognized by acupuncturists as energy meridians. While these meridians have no correspondence to anything in Western medicine, some researchers have established that, in fact, there is a difference in the normal electrical current of the body at the acupuncture points. [157]

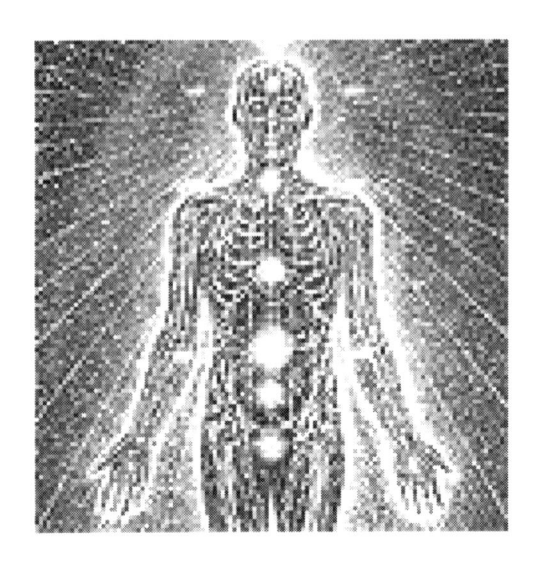

The energy channels as depicted by Alex Grey in his
Energy Anatomy series.

According to the ancient teachings of Indo-Tibetan meditation science, there are at least 72,000 major and minor energy channels in the body. These include the centeral channel, along the spinal column, as well as subtle extensions, some of which come into and go out of existence quickly as part of the mass dynamic of the whole energy body system.

The creative impulse for this network is in what's called the *bindu*, which is described by Fremantle as "the seed point that contains the whole of existence and spreads out infinitely to pervade and encompass the expanse of space".[158] She says it is "...the basic nature of our mind and the essence of life, a continuity of luminous awareness."[159]

> Mind and *bindu* are very closely related, with *bindu* as the basis or instigator of all the different kinds of consciousness. Mind is the creator of everything... but bindu is the creative spark... Mind or consciousness observes, watches what is going on, and responds to it. Bindus pervade the subtle body; they are carried around by prana and they gather in the chakras where they cause the different modes of consciousness to arise.[160]

Being the creative point, the *bindu*, translated as "seed point" or "seed essence", is also used to refer to the sexual essence in men and women. In Tibetan, it's translated as *thigle*, which is described in some detail in the Appendix A of this book.

Through centuries of experience, Tibetan and Indian masters have found and described numerous subtle energy aspects of the nervous and endocrine systems. According to the western-trained Dharma Singh Khalsa, MD, these correspondences have been

> ...verified by the use of sophisticated radioactive scanning methods. The nadis are formed by fine threads of subtle energetic matter... Nadis are an extensive network of fluid-like [energy ducts] which parallel the body nerves in their abundance. The nadis are interwoven with the physical energy system—in intricate interconnection—affecting the nature and quality of nerve transmission within the extensive network of the central nervous system.[161]

In other words, the liquid crystal structures of the material body tissue and the energy transmission structures of the energetic body are indeed one and the same.

The central energy channel is most often spoken of in its association with two parallel "side channels," making up three main vertical energy channels.

> The three main nadis are connected to the brain's limbic system, which controls memory and emotion. It also coordinates the functions of the hypothalamus, and helps control the endocrine's master gland, the pituitary... a tremendously important effect on the body's biochemistry.[162]

These energy channels appear to physically affect the nature and quality of nerve transmission from the brain and spinal cord to the outlying peripheral nerves.

This closely woven interconnection explains why any disturbance of the structure of, or dysfunction in, the chakras and energy channels can impair body function. It can result in quantitative and qualitative dysfunction of the subtle energetic flow to the material body, and, via the hormonal link, can create abnormalities. Such dysfunction precedes and is associated with pathological changes in the nervous and endocrine systems—leading to a variety of disorders.

For example, a decreased flow of energy through the nadis to the throat chakra might result in decreased energy to the thyroid. According to Khalsa, the physical manifestation of this might be hypothyroidism.[163]

Biophysics: Biophotons and the Energy-Body

One of the more exciting developments in the world of science is the integration of the theory and practice of physics with the study of biological systems. As physicists look at cells and tissues, they see things that biologists could not—offering new understandings in the process.

The underlying substance of the universe, the "quantum field of potential," can be understood as a matrix out of which subatomic units sometimes show up as waves of energy and sometimes as particles of matter. These units have been called "wavicles" by quantum physicists and they interact in patterns of vibration that we perceive as the universe—and our bodies.[164]

The most common of these wavicles is the photon, the basic unit of light, which in normal life we experience as a ray or field of light or as a laser beam, and sometimes as a particle hitting, for instance, a computer or television screen. Now, as the structures that make up the human body are analyzed and understood using today's technologies, it's becoming clear that living cells, tissue, and organs appear to generate, and communicate through, light fields and beams—along with other electrochemical signals and fields.

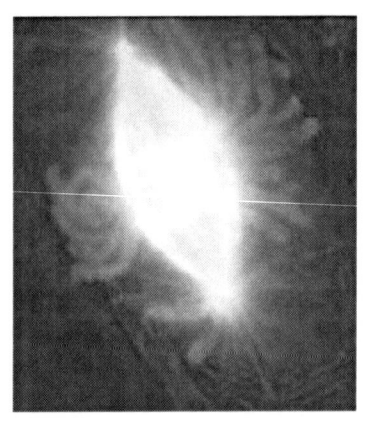

Light emission during cell division.

New Understandings of the Body

Quantum physicist Herbert Frölich demonstrated in the 1970s that living tissue, when "pumped up" with high levels of energy, emits light. Fritz Popp went on to explore many different aspects of this phenomenon. From his work and others we now know that all parts of the living matrix set up vibrations that move about within the organism, and that are radiated into the environment. These vibrations or oscillations occur at many different frequencies, including visible and near visible light.[165]

Dr. Claude Swanson's overview of the physics of subtle energy, *Life Force; The Scientific Basis* gives us a thorough vision of the human body as a biophotonic body, sustained and run by a universal life force which, as we explore earlier, has been called *lung, prana, Ki, reiki,* and *chi,* calling it also bioplasma or torsion.

According to Swanson, this subtle energy is the fifth force in the body and underlies and runs the biophotonic activity of the body.

> Biophotons are quantized packets of light generated in the DNA and other large molecules in the body. The energy they produce is "coherent"... the waves tend to vibrate in step with one another, just like light in a laser. This gives each photon more power, because it is reinforced by the waves of other photons. When waves vibrate in step with one another, they add together to create an interference pattern, a hologram. It is a 3-dimensional pattern of energy which serves as the template of the body...
>
> They communicate it to other DNA molecules in other cells throughout the body. Consequently biophotons are central to understanding physiology.[166]

Reviewing the studies that have been conducted for more than two decades on the nature and content of the energy channels of the traditional acupuncture meridian system, Swanson concludes, "There is a flow within the meridians of both large molecules and energy."[167]

> This explains how a coherent hologram of biophotons arises and generates a coherent torsion [spiral-shaped] field around the body (auric field). Torsion waves have a holographic structure and can maintain patterns of torsion well outside the body.[168]

Again, this concept is not new, even though the direct observation through modern technological enhancements is. In many shamanic traditions, the true self is understood to be a "light body." In Judeo-

Christian traditions, light is synonymous with wisdom, life, and divine power; those who are "filled with light" are healthy and wise and able to guide others in their spiritual life. In Buddhism our fundamental nature is known to be "clear light." It's our potential.

What is "clear light"? Buddhist texts say that it's the radiant luminosity of the ground of being (which we might say is the quantum field out of which matter and energy emerge), and it's obstructed by ordinary consciousness.

According to these texts, the great luminosity of the basis of life is revealed to everyone at the moment before death, when the tendencies of this lifetime have all dissolved.. If they have practiced meditation during their lifetime they will, to some degree, recognize the clear light as their own nature. Otherwise it isn't recognized.[169] The clear light may also manifest in orgasm, and sometimes even in sneezing (which some cultures call "the little death"), but it's rarely recognized.[170]

Dr. Pei-Chen Lo, of the National Chiao Tung University in Taiwan, decided to test the validity of these ancient references. Using the electroencephalogram (EEG), he found that:

> Zen-Buddhist practitioners have discovered that the inner energy is the resource of health and bliss. According to our investigation, the practitioners through years of Zen-Buddhist practice can change the constitution of their bodies by igniting the inner energy. A large number of practitioners are found not only to maintain better health but to remain younger and more energetic than normal people do.[171]

Lo states that

> the spiritual chi can be transformed, via orthodox Zen Buddhist meditation practice, into electrical chi and even light chi that is finally the light of eternal life.[172]

He concludes that the more someone experiences his or her inner light through training and practice, the more he or she will experience enhanced health.

Methods with long proven effects such as *Bum Chung* (offered in Part IV as "Vase Breathing") operate on this model. As described by G. C. C. Chang, *Bum Chung* brings in the subtle energy of vitality by intentionally breathing life energy (lung/prana/chi) into the central energy channel, simultaneously shifting one's focus from the mind-body experience to the larger field of awareness.[173]

With this new information, then, we can state that the human mind-body system is:

> a network of energy flows supporting a network of biochemical flows in the form of body tissue. Maintenance of these energy flows, through the liquid crystals of the body, the chakras, and nadis, governs the wellbeing of the endocrine system, which is the source of the "molecules of emotion" that govern cell activity, and is therefore crucial for the health of the mind-body system.

These flows can be maintained most effectively through the practice of meditation, which is why meditation produces the results described in earlier chapters.

Energy Flows & Fields

In current scientific understanding, atoms and molecules are seen not as solid structures—not little balls revolving around other little balls—but as a dynamic result of the interactions of fields of forces. Atoms are now known to be largely open space, made up of "clouds" or "fields" of positive and negative energy, rather than objects spinning around. These fields form atoms through their constant interaction in a cosmic balancing act. (For some interesting, readable explanations of this phenomenon, try Danah Zohar, *The Quantum Self*, Amit Goswami's *The Self-Aware Universe*, or anything by Fred Alan Wolf.) It was this understanding that led Deepak Chopra to write *Quantum Healing*.

More and more, Westerners are discovering that our experience of the body as static matter is simply a function of our conditioning.

The shamanic traditions and higher initiations of many other cultures lead individuals who are open to the mystery of a different, energy-based reality into a new experience of the body, giving them the ability to see people, animals, and plants as interacting fields of a kind of energy. In her *Hands of Light*, energy healer Barbara Brennan explains her experience in a similar way:

> "The Human Energy Field... can be described as a luminous body that surrounds and interpenetrates the physical body,

emits its own characteristic radiation, and is usually called the "aura".[174]

From the Amazon to Africa and across Asia, new sources of wisdom are being discovered by western scientists that support this model. It was the discovery of this understanding in the mystical traditions that led physicist Fritjof Capra to write his seminal work, *The Tao of Physics*, launched the work of Ken Wilber, and later inspired the movie, *What the Bleep Do We Know?*

The ongoing quantum-mechanical activity that all fields of science are beginning to work with can be understood as patterns of vibration, sometimes in the particle form of matter and sometimes in the wave form of energy. In particle form, the atomic substance of which we are composed is located in a particular point of space and time, with the density of matter. In wave form, the same substance cannot be located, because it's everywhere in space and time.

> an atom... occupies two distinct states, so many times a second... Our matter is blinking on and off... constituted by a rapid succession of instantaneous events... Our bodies are oscillators... we expand into a space-like dimension many times a second... and collapse back as rapidly.[175]

Energy, being the always-moving wave form of subatomic substance, is not fixed in time and space (this is the essence of what's called Heisenberg's Uncertainty Principle). Though it's often portrayed as something like the rings of water that emanate from a pebble striking the surface of a pond, energy is not rays moving across space, but rather *fills* space—in all directions at once. For example, we turn on a light and it fills the room.

The same is true with the energy of our bodies. It exists as fields, partly contained within the tissue and bone. This means that the fields of energy that we are can't be understood as limited to the body. Like all fields of energy, the fields of energy that we are can't be limited by space or time. And the fields of energy that we are interact to create a variety of new, resonating patterns of possibility.

The stability of these fields—being, as are all living systems, dissipative structures—is a function of the continual flow of energy through them, which is evident in the rhythms, the patterns of vibration, which they share. We can see some of these patterns in

New Understandings of the Body

electroencephalograms (EEGs), in electrocardiograms (EKGs), and in magnetic resonance imaging scanners (MRIs). But there's more.

Dr. Karl Maret, one of the researchers exploring these new perceptions, has found that:

> All living processes in the body depend on the transfer of charges to conduct energy and support life. The entire watery matrix of our bodies is interconnected by complex charge-coupled fields that receive about sixty pulsations of electromagnetic energy from our beating heart each minute.... Every cell in the body is in intimate electromagnetic contact with the toroidal-shaped magnetic field of the heart.[176]

Maret observes that the body's heart rate variability provides an instantaneous measure of our entire autonomic nervous system function. It represents essentially the balance between our sympathetic nervous system stress response and the parasympathetic nervous system that is measured in the relaxation response.[177]

And James Oschman tells us:

> The heart beat and all the muscles in the body produce electromagnetic fields, active inside the body and in space. The body's vibrations and oscillations act in many frequencies, internally and externally.... Every muscle in the body produces magnetic pulses when it contracts. The large muscles produce larger fields and the smaller muscles, such as those that move and focus the eye, produce very tiny fields... The fields of all the organs spread throughout the body and into the space around it.[178]

Thus, contrary to the usual medical model of the body as a set of replaceable material-mechanical structures, the human body is now most effectively understood as a set of interacting fields of energy, across the electromagnetic spectrum, and filling the universe.

Oschman expresses this beautifully in *Energy Medicine: The Scientific Basis:*

> On the basis of what is now known about the roles of electrical, magnetic, elastic, acoustic, thermal, gravitational, and photonic energies in human systems, it appears that there... are many energetic systems in the living body, and many ways of

influencing those systems, both known and unknown, functioning collectively, cooperatively, synergistically.

The debate about whether there is such a thing as a healing energy or life force is being replaced with the study of the interactions between biological energy fields, structures and functions.[179]

And again, this understanding, while the result of the most modern physical and biophysical investigation, is also an ancient one, with variations in cultures ranging from Tibet to Mexico, Siberia to Australia. For example, in *The Active Side of Infinity*, a Yaqui shaman shared the ancient teachings of this tradition by asserting:

> ...when a human being is *seen*, he is perceived as a conglomerate of energy fields held together by the most mysterious force in the universe: a binding, agglutinating, vibratory force that holds energy fields together in a cohesive unit.[180]

Resonant Fields: Mind-Body Energy in Context

As a pattern of subtle energy forming a unique set of interactive energy fields, the mind-body functions within a larger set of interactive fields.

This pattern we are is easily influenced, yet remarkably stable, as it encounters these other energy forms.

> Our biological rhythms are entrained by light and to a certain extent by gravitational effects... magnetic, electromagnetic, atmospheric, and subtle geophysical effects influence us... Our mind-body is resonant with these rhythmically entrained field effects, natural and man-made. We're also surrounded and permeated by the static electricity field and by the electrostatic fields created by our body.[181]

That includes the fields that compose and surround the Earth. Many of these larger fields are measurable on the electromagnetic spectrum and their activity is observed through a variety of technologies.

The electromagnetic fields around the Earth affect us in several ways. Our planet is surrounded by a moving layer of electrically charged particles called the ionosphere. The Earth is made up of water and minerals that are predominantly negatively charged. The

New Understandings of the Body

ionosphere is positively charged. So there's a difference in electrical potential between the two. The resulting structure is what is called a magnetosphere, a field of electrical activity around a metal core, which is, in fact, a type of electrical generator. We know this partly because we can see and measure electrically charged streams from the Sun, called solar winds, interacting with the rotating upper atmosphere like the brushes of an electrical generator, making the beautiful glow we call the "aurora."

The lower atmosphere, another field, located between the Earth and the ionosphere, acts like a storage battery for the electrical potential that is built up between them. Observing this in the 1950s, German geophysicist Dr. W. O. Schumann suggested that electromagnetic signals circulate at extremely low frequencies between the Earth and the ionosphere. These signals came to be called "Schumann's Resonances" (SR) and, it turns out, the frequencies of these SR signals increase or decrease with ionospheric conditions, which change daily, seasonally, with the lunar cycle, and with variations in solar activity.

So long as the properties of Earth's electromagnetic cavity remain about the same, these frequencies remain the same. They seem to be related only to electrical activity in the atmosphere, particularly during times of intense lightning activity. There's no evidence suggesting that they're caused by terrestrial factors like Earth's tectonic plate movements or even shifts in the Earth's core, even though those features also produce magnetic fields.

Like waves on the ocean or on a stringed musical instrument, SR must be potentiated or "excited" to be observed. They've been observed in experiments occurring at several harmonic frequencies.

Not too surprisingly, since we evolved as part of this terrestrial electrical system, these frequencies are the same cycles as the typical theta (sleep) and beta (waking state) brainwave rhythms documented on EEGs, and the blank range between the first two levels is a very reasonable match with the alpha (dreaming and light meditation) rhythm. The planet, it seems, exhibits the same states of consciousness as we do!

In their exploration of these ideas, Richard and Iona Miller tell us:

> Schumann's resonance forms a natural feedback loop with the human mind/body. The human brain and body developed in

the biosphere, the [electromagnetic] environment conditioned by this cyclic pulse. Conversely, this pulse acts as a "driver" of our brains and can also potentially carry information. Functional processes may be altered and new patterns of behavior facilitated through the brain's web of inhibitory and excitatory feedback networks.[182]

They also suggest that, because oscillating patterns tend to set up resonance with other oscillating patterns, changes in Schumann's Resonances may lead to changes in the pattern of oscillation in our individual electromagnetic fields, and, conversely, the oscillation pattern of any individual may affect the patterns of those around that person and the larger field, as well.

Apparently the frequency of these resonances has been changing over the past several years. Now, in 2012, rather than paralleling our own internal rhythms, the SR frequencies are reported on various websites to be almost double what they were 50 years ago. This may be a result of increasing temperature in the ionosphere or it may be a response to increased solar activity. In any case, to the extent that the mind-body will tend to resonate with the field around it, the change is likely affecting human experience.[183]

Morphic Resonance & Collective Consciousness

Rupert Sheldrake is an evolutionary biologist who sought to understand how it is that similar mutations in plants and animals have occurred across the planet at very nearly the same time without direct interaction. In his ground breaking book, *A New Science of Life*, Sheldrake offers a number of related examples and proposed a "Theory of Morphic Resonance" to explain them. He hypothesizes that the occurrence of an event anywhere increases the likelihood of the same event happening everywhere and calls the mechanism by which this might occur "resonating morphogenetic fields".[184]

> There's a hierarchy of fields organizing the body. There's the field of the whole organism, the fields of our organs, the fields of our tissues and of the cells within those. The fields of our body include subsidiary fields, moderating fields and then those of arms, legs, and the different organs. [185]

Such fields, "have the advantage of being holistic… if you cut up a magnet, into however many little bits… each has a complete magnetid field."[186] Body fields, being morphogenetic fields, he says, are not physical in the sense of being measurable by the usual electromagnetic devices, but they are more like resonating patterns of information encompassing the organism and the planet, which, when a life form resonates with it, generates a new internal and external form for that life.

> ...morphogenetic fields differ radically from electromagnetic fields in that the latter depend on the... distribution and movement of charged particles —whereas morphogenetic fields correspond to the potential state of a developing system and are already present before it takes up its final form.[187]

The morphogenetic field is in place before the matter-energy takes form! It is, in fact, the mould, the template, that determines the form that the matter-energy will take. An example from human experience would be the process by which a secret scientific discovery occurs in one laboratory and is often repeated almost immediately several times in other places, long before anyone outside of the original laboratory knows about the first discovery.

One of Sheldrake's examples suggesting Morphic Resonance occurred many years before he proposed his theory. Generations of rats were trained to do a new task at Harvard, in Massachusetts. Some time later, a different group of rats were trained to do the same task in Edinburgh. The Edinburgh group learned the task far more quickly—some without even being trained.[188]

An intriguing aspect of this theory is its similarity to the model of human consciousness suggested by Carl Jung. In Jung's model, individual consciousness is seen as an open-ended field within a larger field, the collective consciousness.

As presented by Oliver W Markley and Willis Harman in *Changing Images of Man*[189] the collective field is divided into the collective subconscious, associated with the darker emotions, fear, and attachment to matter, and the collective superconscious, associated with high ideals and values. Jung hypothesized that ideas and forms present in dreams and stories across cultures (archetypes) are located in this collective consciousness, accessible to and affecting the individual's awareness as the individual is ready to experience them— or, using Sheldrake's term, resonates with them.

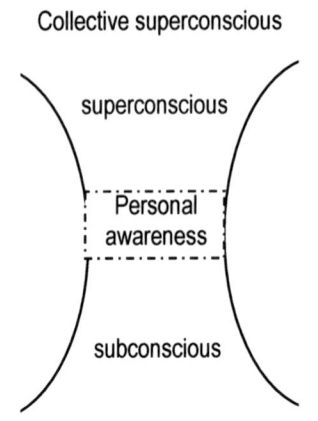

```
        Collective superconscious

              superconscious

              ┌─────────────┐
              │  Personal   │
              │  awareness  │
              └─────────────┘

              subconscious

        Collective subconscious
```

The Morphic Resonance and Collective Consciousness theories were developed apart from Schumann's work with atmospheric resonance, but both of them support and extend it. If, as the Millers have suggested, the electromagnetic oscillation pattern within the atmospheric cavity can carry information (which we know is true because that is exactly how radio works), then both archetypal structures and new insights or mutations could well be encoded in the resonant pattern of Earth's electromagnetic field.

The patterns of information would therefore be instantaneously available to any resonating energy pattern anywhere on the planet, just as a radio, tuned to the right frequency, can receive information almost as it is transmitted. Transpersonal interaction must therefore be considered an integral part of the human mind-body.

A Negentropic Holographic System

Taking these ideas together, we can see that the mind-body is a living system with all the characteristics of such systems. It's a complex structure of matter, energy, and information working to maintain itself, which it does by continuously (in cycles of growth and rest) increasing in complexity. It's dependent on consistent flows of energy, which it can accept in the form of matter, light and other forms of energy, or as information. It functions as a whole: every part is physically and psychologically interconnected with, and affected by, every other part.

New Understandings of the Body

As we've seen, hese tendencies—to take in matter, energy, and information in any form and convert it to physical energy, to increase in complexity, and to function as a whole—are what distinguish living systems from other forms of systems. Because of them, living systems are, in fact, negentropic.

These tendencies are also the key to understanding the healing process. To the extent that a healing modality addresses them, it will be effective and cause no harm. In fact, it will enhance these tendencies and encourage the system's ongoing development. And meditation, in all its forms, is such a modality.

They also suggest that the mind-body system is not the material body that we see and measure, but that the measurable, material body is what's called an "emergent property" of the system: it's the result, rather than the cause, of the various patterns of energy and information we've been describing. Maret and others have observed communication via coherent light within and among cells and suggested that this permits the holistic functioning of the body, because it's identical to the way holograms are made. We're suggesting that it's the other way around: the cells *are* the hologram and the biophotons are the means by which we can perceive them.

The Multiple Bodies of the Human Mind-Body

As we consider our usual experience of muscle, bone, and organs in the context of our intuitive and imaginative thinking and emotional experience—quite apart from what modern science has told us about energy fields—we find it impossible not to perceive several "bodies" as our own. Yet, though common in human experience, this is not an understanding common in the Western scientific tradition. We would be hard put to find the language to describe how such a body works and can be assisted if we were only able to look there. Fortunately, when we allow for the possibility that other traditions may equally inform our understanding, we find the idea to be not only present, but fundamental, as we will explore in the following pages.

The Western Spiritual Model

Although the religious traditions of the West have not been built on a scientific paradigm, nor even a psychology of consciousness, there are elements of a multi-body model of human experience expressed in both the sacred literature and daily practice of Judaism, Christianity, and Islam (collectively, the Abramic traditions) that should not be ignored in our search for a working model of the mind-body.

Within these traditions each individual consists of a soul and a body and is physically and spiritually isolated from all others except, possibly, at some distant time, God. The body is considered to be a temporary physical and emotional construct based on the experiences and expressions of the individual. The soul, while not fully integrated with the body, is understood to be the life force of the body, existing before and after the body, and affected by the body's experiences and expressions—its destiny being determined, in large part, by them. This split between the body and the soul is fundamental to the practices and principles of all three traditions. It's what permits Muslim "suicide bombers" to feel good about what they do and is what drove the Catholic Church to "save souls" without regard to the state of the body for the many years of colonization, the Inquisition, and the witch hunts.[190]

A third element, called Spirit, enters into the picture with the New Testament. It originally referred to what Jesus called "the Comforter" and was experienced as a wind and a flame at Pentecost. The apostle Paul, exhorting his followers not to "walk in the way of the flesh" but of Spirit (in Romans 7 and 8 et al.) and encouraging them to develop "gifts of the Spirit" (in I Corinthians et al.), shifted the original concept from an experience to a state of being. The current idea is that, through God's good grace and no effort or special deserving by the individual, "the Holy Spirit enters in" to some people and transforms them, providing gifts such as prophecy and healing. It's a central element of the Pentecostal Christian movement, charismatic Catholicism, and many of the fundamentalist Protestant doctrines.

In metaphysical New Thought churches, the Holy Spirit is understood to be the omnipresent essence of all that is, formless yet expressing through and as each being. Rather than being a "gift" from somewhere "outside" our world, it is the "essence" or "true nature" of each individual. And the soul, then, is the result of the interaction between the Spirit and the body.

The "Christ mind," which the apostle Paul exhorted his followers to "let be in your mind" (in Philippians 2) adds another dimension to

New Understandings of the Body

the Christian model. He defined this mind as a way of being that exhibits no human judgment, offering only compassion, unconditional love, and acceptance. In traditional Christianity, this is a discipline, achieved by study and prayer, and recently, by following the maxim "What Would Jesus Do?" In the metaphysical New Thought churches, this is considered a state of consciousness, called Christ Consciousness, that can be attained through study, prayer, meditation, and repeated affirmation of the intention.

This model becomes more complex with the integration of "spiritualist" Judaism and Christianity into the picture. In this centuries-old tradition, Jesus and the prophets are understood to have conversed with people who have "passed on" and are no longer in physical form (for example, the disciples' observation of Jesus' conversation with Moses and Elijah in the story called "The Transfiguration"), and so modeled for their followers that they should do likewise. Spiritualist churches therefore include channeling of messages from "the other side" in their otherwise traditional Christian services. This idea of the spirit as separate from soul and body is also seen in what is known as "voodoo," which includes many related rituals in otherwise Christian services. The idea of the individual spirit is sometimes confused with the biblical concept of soul, because both exist before and after this lifetime, but they are seen as separate in this model.

In the mid-19th century, with the first translations of sacred texts from the East, a new model emerged within the Christian tradition: the Transcendentalists. Ralph Waldo Emerson, Henry David Thoreau, Walt Whitman, Margaret Fuller, and the Alcotts were instrumental in bringing into popular American awareness the fundamental ideas of this movement. These include: the possibility of a direct perception of reality, unmediated by thought; a unification with mankind and Nature; an identification with the divine as an Oversoul that includes all beings; and a way of thinking, speaking, and acting that transcends social norms and expectations.

One significant development out of the Transcendentalist movement was the application of these ideas in Christian Science and the New Thought tradition. Both Christian Science and the New Thought tradition see the body as the manifestation of all of the beliefs, thoughts, ideas, and expectations held in mind, the individual mind as a part of a universal Mind of God, and the individual soul or spirit as part of the eternal, omnipresent Spirit of God.[191]

The Western Esoteric Model

Polls over the past several decades tell us that from around 50% to more than 80% of Americans acknowledge having "mystical" experiences. Some of the reported experiences include seeing "ghosts" and feeling, smelling, or hearing invisible presences; seeing or hearing a nonmaterial being acting to guard or protect one; observing things or beings appear or disappear in inexplicable ways; unexplained healings and remissions of disease; and direct visual or oral communications with people who are known to be elsewhere or dead. (This will not surprise regular listeners of the popular nighttime radio talk show *Coast to Coast AM*!) A large body of literature has emerged over the past two centuries exploring these experiences, through which it's become clear that the materialist-scientific tradition can't, and traditional religion has not been willing to, explain them.

The lack of religious (outside of Spiritualist churches) or scientific explanations for these experiences in the nineteenth and early twentieth centuries led a few scientifically minded people to rigorously investigate such experiences, which in turn led to the formation of the British Society for Psychical Research, the Theosophical Society, and several other associations seeking to understand scientifically what was explained by neither science nor religion. The reports of rigorous tests in the journals and books produced by these associations and their members are numerous and exhaustive.

One summary of these texts is *The Basic Ideas of Occult Wisdom* by Anne Kennedy Winner. She says:

> We are told that every human body, besides the dense physical core which we see, has in it and around it a number of interpenetrating sheaths (sheath in the sense of container...) ... every man has an "etheric" or "vital" sheath or body, which is physical in the sense of belonging to the physical plane, and in being discarded at death, but which is invisible to ordinary sight, because it is made up of "matter" of the finest or "etheric" subdivisions of the physical plane... a kind of "force field" which

forms the matrix or energy pattern upon which the dense physical form is built... [192]

In *The Doctrine of the Subtle Body in Western Tradition*, G. R. S. Mead explores the various understandings of spirit, ethereal body, subtle body, and related concepts throughout Western history. Drawing on the writings of minds as diverse as Plato and Tertullian, Aristotle and Menander, Mead summarizes dozens of conceptualizations of the human being as consisting of something more than a material body, having something variously termed a "spirit," a "subtle body," a "soul," and a "resurrection body."

Together, these writings point to a model of the human being in which an eternal essence takes form in two stages: as spirit or subtle body and then as material body. Then, through imagination, thought, word, and activity, the two together facilitate the subtle body's return to the eternal, and the material body is either discarded or resurrected in union with the spirit/subtle body.

Western Alternative Healing Traditions

In *Vibrational Medicine*, Richard Gerber MD, integrates a model of the human mind-body structure from a variety of energy-healing traditions. His model describes five inseparable bodies: the physical body, a mental body, an astral body, an etheric body, and a causal body. This multifold body model permits different levels and types of activity and explains the different types of human experience.

According to Gerber's integration of these models, the physical body is the material, manifest body that interacts with the material world around it. The mental body is the field of energy that is formed by and forms one's thoughts and logical reasoning and so affects the functioning of the material body.

Gerber states that the astral body is composed of a substance that is neither matter nor energy (perhaps the quantum field?) and so is not limited by the laws of matter, but can function in the material world as well as on what is called "the astral plane," a dimension of existence that is very dream like and is, according to many, where much of our dream work happens. (Being built on emotions and irrational feelings, the astral body has a profound impact on the material body and is the body form of most "ghosts", which may be understood as beings whose life experiences were so intense that they have been unable to leave the situation of the experiences.)

The etheric body, Gerber says, is almost pure energy and corresponds to the unique self, or spirit, of the individual. Like the astral body, it transcends space and time, but it is pure awareness, free of the intense emotions that drive and form the astral body.

Finally, he says, the causal body is that aspect of self that experiences this lifetime as part of an eternal experience and carries into this lifetime memories and understandings from other lifetimes. It's sometimes referred to as the Higher Self.

> The etheric and physical bodies, being of different frequencies, overlap and coexist within the same space... Energy disturbances in the etheric body and the acupuncture meridian system precede the physical/cellular manifestation of illness.... The astral body is... made up of matter of a higher frequency than etheric matter. It is similarly superimposed upon the physical-etheric framework.... Consciousness can move into the astral body and separate from the physical and etheric vehicles. When this occurs naturally it is known as astral projection or an Out-Of-Body Experience (OOBE). When this separation of consciousness occurs traumatically it is often referred to as a Near Death Experience (NDE)...[193]

In Gerber's model every moment of human existence is experienced through the interaction of these bodies. Development of individuals is seen as the capacity to identify and choose which body one is operating from at any time. We gradually move from the physical and astral bodies through the mental to the causal and etheric, or eternal/celestial essence. But we're never in one body at a time. The bodies that we're developing are dynamically interresonant at all times.

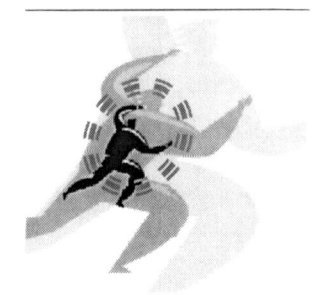

Multiple bodies working together; decreasing in density while increasing in energy and space.

New Understandings of the Body

Ultimately, Gerber tells us, one aims to be aware of all of them all the time and to act in ways that ensure harmony at all levels.

The Upanishads

Perhaps the most ancient documented scientific research may be found in the Hindu Upanishads, written in Sanskrit somewhere between 3,000 and 4,000 years ago. Buddhist researchers working in the past millennium knew the models presented in these ancient texts and incorporated many of the concepts into their own frameworks.

One of these is the idea of a subtle body inseparable from the physical body, with a threefold nature, described in Sanskrit: *nadi, prana,* and *bindu*. In this model, *nadi*, which means "river", or "channel," or "tube", refers to the extensive network of energy channels described earlier in this chapter. They form the structure of the subtle body, the energy body. The network of nadis can be imagined as channels through which *prana* flows, life energy sustaining the physical body. The channels are formed by the force of what's called the pranic flow.

In the Upanishads this pranic body is described as:

> ...a second body within the physical body called the "vital body" or "vital sheath." ...the physical body is nothing more than a crystallization around the energy pattern that underlies it.[194]

The Three-Body Buddhist Model

The Buddhist description of the *Trikaya*, "the three bodies," offers another compelling model of the multidimensional nature of humanity. Having emerged from the Vedic tradition, Buddhists use Sanskrit terms for these aspects of being: *Dharmakaya, Sambhogakaya,* and *Nirmanakaya*. Francesca Fremantle, in her book *Luminous Emptiness*, describes the *trikaya* as "the threefold pattern of the awakened state," stating that Chogyam Trungpa used to speak of it as the pattern of life in general.

Dharmakaya means "truth body" or "body of absolute nature." Psychologically this is defined as the empty or open nature of the body, inseparable from pure awareness. Physically it can be defined as the quantum field within the atomic nature of the corporal form, the subatomic void of pure potential, from which the universe and its infinite forms emerge. The Dharmakaya is the nonlocal, universal field, the basis of the human being's unlimited nature, the person's timeless, deathless nature. The Dharmakaya may correspond to what Georges Gurdjieff called essence, the fundamental nature of being. It's what physicist Amit Goswami calls the consciousness that pervades and creates the material world.[195]

Spontaneously arising from the Dharmakaya is the *Sambhogakaya*, which is the connecting form, the body of light, the body of communication. Fremantle describes it in terms of light:

> Light radiates from the emptiness of dharmakaya as the five colors of the five kinds of knowledge. It appears in shining rainbow clouds, in glowing circles, in scintillating pinpoints, and dazzling rays of light. Then the five colors crystallize into... divine forms... made entirely of light; they arise out of light and dissolve back into light. This is the realm of sacred vision... the bridge between emptiness and form: emptiness displaying itself as form; form revealing itself to be emptiness. [196]

In Buddhist meditation Sambhogakaya is a radiant form within the material body, the visionary form of what's often called deity nature. Visualizing this form can be understood as a practice of seeing our sacred energy body as the body of our potential. As Fremantle puts it:

> The experience of the sambhogakaya is to perceive the world directly and nakedly, welcoming whatever appears without preconceptions. Sense perceptions become clearer, sharper, and more colorful.... The world is recognized as sacred, magical, and full of wonder. It contains all the vitality and passion of the emotions, free from the confusion that brings misery and pain.[197]

One focuses on this radiant "bridge between emptiness and form," this inner light, in order to:

- communicate with the unlimited potential of the Dharmakaya within
- practice the wisdom and power of the light nature of embodiment, the Sambhogakaya, radiating wellbeing into all aspects of life
- not lose our true nature by identifying only with the manifest nature, the Nirmanakaya

- restore balance and set body, mind, and spirit in primal order
- thus restore health and access our inherent potential.

The *Nirmanakaya*, or manifest nature, is the actual physical body energy appearing as matter, to act in the realm of matter. The term literally means "body of emanation" because it emanates from the Sambhogakaya. It is sometimes called "the causal body." In its highest form, it is the embodiment of the energy of compassion and totally responsive to the needs of all beings. The Tibetan term for this highest form is *Tulku*, a title given to one who is recognized as a great teacher reborn with full awareness of his or her Buddha-nature and with the conscious intention to benefit others. However, as Fremantle reminds us, "we are all really nirmanakaya, but we do not realize it".[198]

The Buddhist model, therefore, places the material body in a matrix of universality (Dharmakaya) and radiant divinity (Sambhogakaya), and emerges as an expression and experience of both. With this model, all of life's processes can be seen as movement within and among these three aspects of being, and focusing on the radiant light nature of the Sambhogakaya becomes a means for bringing a higher order of functioning to our physical nature. Fremantle says:

> The experience of the *trikaya* can be found everywhere; it is a continual presence in our lives. The *dharmakaya* is present in the sense of openness, the source and background of all phenomena. The *sambhogakaya* is present in the sense of energy bursting forth, the sacred, magical quality of life. And the *nirmanakaya* is present in the sense of phenomena continually arising, impermanent yet vividly apparent.[199]

Within this threefold body structure, Buddhist research says that each sentient being has three "doors"—body, speech, and mind—through which our deeds, thoughts, and words work in the world. Body refers to the manifest, material form and corresponds to the Nirmanakaya. "It is the outward expression in material form of our mind and energy."[200] Speech corresponds to Sambhogakaya: energy, emotion, and communication. It refers to both the outward sounds and the inner emotions from which they emanate. The invisible, formless mind corresponds to the Dharmakaya, including all our thoughts, perceptions, feelings, and reactions, and encompassing the Western ideas of heart and mind, together.

Fremantle points out that the same tri-fold pattern continues in the Buddhist concept of "coarse, subtle, and very subtle body and mind" saying that these three correspond to "the waking state, the state of dreaming, and the state of deep sleep".[201] The coarse body is the flesh-and-blood-and-bones that we usually think of as our body, including the hormonal and nerve systems that manifest specific states, and corresponds to the Nirmanakaya. The subtle body, or mind-body, like the Sambhogakaya, bridges between our physical experience and pure awareness. The very subtle body is nearly indescribable, corresponding to the emptiness of the Dharmakaya, typically illustrated as the union of the male and female principles in the heart. It is often called the intrinsic Buddha-nature and is the essence of life, "a continuity of luminous awareness".[202]

Integrating Models of the Human Mind-Body

So far we've described various models of the human mind-body that have emerged in history. Now, with the advances in science, technology, anthropology, and psychology described in the previous chapter, it's possible to begin to define a model for the emerging medical paradigm. It's a model that provides a framework for theraperutic mind-body practices in which the full potential of the human mind-body may be realized, allowing new kinds of administered care and for a medicine based on self-care,

In this model mind, body, and spirit are clearly inseparable, and the ancient and most recent ideas are integrated. As a result, it's possible to see how new ways of addressing health challenges may help people realize what human beings truly are and may become.

1. **Mind and body are physically, chemically, and energetically inseparable.**

    As a living system, the mind-body is a complex set of interconnections in delicate balance, such that any small action has a profound effect on every aspect—more so even than a house of cards. Mental and emotional activity have as profound an effect on the whole system as physical activity and chemical input do. And, as with all systems, we can "never do just one thing," so we must be aware of all the secondary and tertiary effects of the actions we take—and the thoughts we think. To treat the mind is to treat the body, and vice versa. Therefore, any healing modality must take all aspects of the individual into consideration if it is to be effective.

2. **That which we call the body is not a solid, fixed object but a dynamic set of interacting energy fields, oscillating in a unique resonant pattern and generating the appearance of matter in the presence of an observer.**

    All that we perceive and measure is not actually solid matter, but a set of resonant fields that appear to us as matter. The more complex a structure or system is, the more fields are involved and the more modes of information exchange and transmission are observed. The human mind-body, therefore, is not just the bundle of nerves, bone, and tissue that we observe—it's a hologram, generated by the oscillation of energies and information exchanged within the set of fields that makes up each individual. And the unique pattern of resonance that holds the fields together defines the individual system, the holographic mind-body that's constantly being generated to match our perceptual senses. Therefore, to change the body, we must change the fields first.

3. **The energy fields of which we are composed and those that we generate range in frequency across the electromagnetic spectrum and beyond, including both perceivable and imperceptible levels of light and other forms of information-organized energy.**

There are a number of technologies used in the medical world and in laboratories that provide visual images of electrical, magnetic, light, and what many call the "etheric" fields of the body. Many more are measuring the various forms of energy generated through interactions of the matter and energy that make up the mind-body system. As scientists begin to accept this interaction as the natural state of the mind-body, they see more and more evidence supporting it. Therefore, the effects of thoughts and emotion, as well as other subtle energy shifts within and around the body, must be considered when physical dysfunction or disease appears.

4. **These fields interact in such a way that cells, tissue, and organs develop and are maintained as the manifest material mind-body, which is called *Nirmanakhaya* in the Buddhist traditions.**

We can see that cells and tissues are best understood as the holographic projection of the fields that sustain them, and those fields are composed of interacting energy and information. Therefore, our focus shifts from the material symptoms to the underlying energy patterns. Discovering and maintaining healthy mental and emotional states, as well as appropriate energy flows and fields within and around the body, is now seen as most useful for achieving and maintaining wellbeing.

5. **The material mind-body is sustained by a continuous flow of energy through the energy fields and cellular structures that constitute it, and it is sustained and potentially increased in force through the negentropic nature of living systems.**

As a dissipative structure, the living system of the mind-body require consistent flows of energy. Light, electrochemical, and more subtle energy flows sustain the mind-body and are influenced by mental activity. This realization leads us to shift our focus from attempting to repair the material body to discovering the mental, emotional, and energetic blocks to the healthy flow of these energies and maintenance of these fields. It also helps us to understand that the mind-body is a continually developing system that doesn't naturally tend to wear down like machines, but rather tends to increase in complexity and elegance. Therefore, healing becomes a process, not of preventing wearing out, but of encouraging development and transformation.

6. **The energy fields, and the material mind-body they sustain, are part of, affect, and are affected by a larger set of energy fields that surround the planet and pervade the solar system, within which are the fields and flows of energy that sustain the mind-body.**

As a living system and dissipative structure, the human mind-body is dependent on near-constant flows of energy to maintain its structure. As part of the larger earth and solar system, its energy fields and flows are intricately connected with their fields and flows. As part of the morphogenetic field of humanity, the structure of the individual mind-body is defined largely by the current collective consciousness of the whole. This means that the electromagnetic fields (often called EMFs) surrounding the earth, as well as our homes and businesses, are in constant interaction with the energy field that each human being is, affecting the overall well-being of the material body. It also means the individual is under constant pressure from the collective consciousness to align with it. Therefore, understanding individual symptoms of disease or distress may depend in part on understanding the larger fields of the collective consciousness and the planet.

7. **Flows and interactions in the energy fields of the mind-body are regulated by the rhythms of the heart; they can be blocked, pulled out of balance, or enhanced, all of which directly affects function in the manifest mind-body.**

Energy fields exist in relation to other fields, not in isolation. How they function is determined by their interaction with other fields (as, for example, the poles of a magnet: opposite poles together are attracting fields; same poles are repulsing fields). This means that the fields that comprise living systems must remain open and in balance for the system to remain healthy. In the realm of animals and humans, this balance is maintained by the electromagnetic pulses associated with the rhythms of the heartbeat. To the extent that our mental and emotional activities harmonize with and maintain the integrity of this rhythm and the energy flows and fields that we are, the mind-body system is balanced and external fields have less disruptive effects. Therefore, an effective healing modality restores balance to those interacting energy flows.

8. **Blocks and imbalances in the material body may emerge through interactions with disruptive energy fields, or through patterns of thought and feeling which introduce information that block or modify flows in the system.**

Thoughts and feelings held in the mind affect the electrical and chemical activity of the body in often unexpected, and too often damaging, ways. Biochemically, powerful stress-inducing thoughts or feelings can shut down immune function, digestion, and blood flows to parts of the body; continuous low-level stressors can hamper the functioning of many subsystems of the body; and joyful, loving experiences can reverse those tendencies. Energetically, long term low-level emotional states can block energy flows with similar results. Clarifying the energy flows can reverse some or all of these tendencies. Therefore, an effective healing modality removes blocks to energy flows within the mind-body system.

9. **The material body is only one aspect of the human mind-body system. A second body, consisting of almost no matter and almost completely energy, has been called the body of radiant communication, the *Sambhogakaya*, the etheric**

body, the celestial body, or spirit.

Although there is little accepted theory in the Western scientific tradition to support this aspect of our model, virtually every culture on the planet has both anecdotal and theoretical support for it. Accepting that the material body is actually a holographic projection supposes that there is an energy-information system projecting the hologram. (To use a *Star Wars* metaphor, there must be an R2D2 projecting Princess Leia's image; or, from *Star Trek, Next Generatioon*, there must be an energy source programmed to project an experience on the holodeck.) This energy-information system projects and maintains the material body as it develops, balancing the individual's mental and emotional activity with the morphogenetic field structure in which it's formed and the energetic flows around and through it. This means that a healing method focused only on the manifest, material body is attempting to repair the projection rather than the projector.

10. There is a universal field potential unique to each being and constantly interacting with all other beings and fields, the *Dharmakaya, Brahman, rigpa,* or Higher Self.

The underlying quantum field, the source of "life energy" or lung/chi/prana, is the source of all matter and energy, and is one interconnected whole, throughout the spacetime continuum of this universe and perhaps beyond. This is the One, the ground of being, the clear light, the transcendent mystery underlying all, of which we are all part and of which we have so little awareness as a human mind-body system. Yet, in some way, some part of us works outside of our normal space and time to generate what Carl Jung called "synchronicities"—experiences that support and encourage our continued development. Some meditators have glimpsed this aspect of being. They do so when their usual emotional and mental activity is silenced, which leads to enhanced flows of energy throughout the mind-body system, increasing overall wellbeing by bringing the system into alignment with the larger field.

Implications Of The Model

The model we are proposing defines the individual mind-body that each of us calls "me" as a unique pattern of interactions among the various aspects of one multifold body, with its heart-centered resonating rhythms, simultaneous with its unique pattern of interaction with the larger system of energy fields and bodies that surround it.

Clearly, this model is a radical departure from the way most of us have been taught to think about our bodies and how they work. Equally clearly, Western scientific medicine as it has evolved cannot provide effective methods for working with this more complete envisioning of the reality of the living human body.

This is no longer Era I medicine, based on a mechanical anatomical model of the physical body learned from dissected corpses. We have entered Era II and Era III medicine, in both cases based on a model of living material body, mind-body, and energy body as inseparable aspects of being.

Fortunately, methods are available now that can work powerfully with this model of the human body—and new mind-body self-care methods are being created and discovered all the time.

∞

A New Model of the Healing Process

As we understand more about the dynamics of the mind-body system, we can see that some of the routine activities of Western "scientific medicine" may create more problems than they solve. As long as the body was seen as a mechanical system run by complex biochemical processes, healing was understood as removing or replacing parts by surgery, and providing the appropriate chemical or combination of chemicals to achieve a desired state. However, as soon as we acknowledge that thought, emotions, and mental imagery play a role in maintaining the mind-body system—on the part of both the patient and the care provider—then a very different description of the healing process becomes necessary.

A new model of healing recognizes the mind-body system as a set of interacting elements sustained by relatively constant energy flows through the system.

Healers working from such a model would not suddenly shift those energy flows, recognizing that too great a fluctuation could result in the collapse of the system. Nor would they expect fixed or constant behaviors on the part of individuals, or even their bodies. Instead, they would recognize a range of possible states as "normal." Static states and continuous movement would be seen as unlikely, at best. Recognizing the complex set of interactions making up the person before them, they would tend to seek a dynamic equilibrium, and they would teach their patients how to achieve and maintain that equilibrium on their own, using empowering self-care methods.

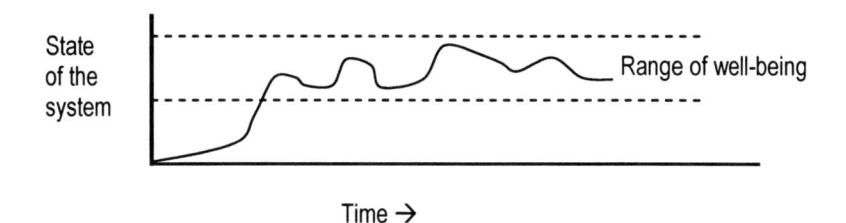

As we understand more clearly the structure of the mind-body, we begin to shift our assumptions and expectations about the nature of its condition. Because the condition of the material body is a function of what is happening in the energy fields and in their interaction with the material body through the many energy channels, seeing the energy body as central to human function becomes a diagnostic and therapeutic tool. Numerous "medical intuitives," such as Jane Katra, coauthor of *Miracles of Mind* and Caroline Myss, as presented in *The Anatomy of the Spirit*, have demonstrated the utility of the energy body model in many situations, and physicians like Norman Shealy and Larry Dossey have learned to rely on such understandings:

Anyone who is aware of the recent trends in medicine will realize that modern physicians—like the physicists before them—have begun to deal with finer and finer forms of energy both in the diagnosis and treatment of human illness.[203]

As we understand more fully the interactive relationship between any individual and the living systems in which that individual acts, we begin to integrate more people into our treatment protocols, and we pay more attention to the interpersonal and transpersonal context in which the individual is functioning.

Illness as a State of Consciousness

As we consider the continuum of states of consciousness in the illustration on p.81 we see that some can be described as "more harmonious" and some as "less harmonious" with regard to the interacting functions of the mind-body system. For example, the states we've labeled Anxiety and Rage are associated with heightened adrenaline release, heart rate, and blood pressure—all of which disturb other physiological functions. They're also associated with limited mental functioning, which reduces the individual's capacity to respond to a changing environment. By contrast, in the state of Alert Rest the full range of mental function is operative and physiological functions are optimized.

Illness results from ongoing dysfunctions in the mind-body system that shift the body's normal responses to challenges to the point where they're no longer sufficient to maintain healthy function. It's associated with physiological functions that are other than healthy, and to the extent that the person experiencing it is

A New Model of the Healing Process

experiencing emotions of distress, illness is clearly a "less harmonious" state of being. Therefore, to the extent that the body is, like all other forms, a projection of mind—the particular thoughts, emotions, beliefs, and assumptions held by the individual—the state of being we call illness must be understood as a state of consciousness.

Looking at illness this way, we can identify a number of generic characteristics that apply almost regardless of the particular symptoms. The person experiencing the state of illness:

- experiences body sensations acutely
- experiences challenges in multiple aspects of functioning
- has unique, more-frequent-than-normal periods of sleep and dreaming
- is more passive than active
- is freed from normal behavioral and reactive patterns

These characteristics apply to every experience of illness, in whatever form. They may be the defining characteristics of this particular state of consciousness.

This suggests that the way out of the experience of illness is to change one's state of consciousness. And this understanding is exactly what Quimby, Eddy, Hopkins, and thousands of shamans "mental healers" and "faith healers" have worked with through the millennia.[204] They have treated the consciousness of the individual rather than the symptoms of the body. They have focused on restoring balance in the mind-body system rather than on "fixing" a particular structure or function in the body. As they've done so, some of their patients' lives have been transformed: they longer functioned in the same way. In the depths of the state of consciousness of illness they found spirit to heal body and mind, and so experienced a new way of living.

Illness, then, like all states of consciousness, has its opportunities as well as challenges. Because of those opportunities, illness may be understood as a process through which transformation becomes possible. With this book, we hope to identify the essential processes and methods that disclose the opportunities and make the inherent potential for transformation a reality.

Transpersonal Medicine

In his comprehensive study entitled *Transpersonal Medicine*, Frank Lawlis, a medical doctor trained in traditional, allopathic institutions, has done an excellent job of identifying the major concerns and contributions in the field, starting with the proposition that,

> ...at its root, transpersonal medicine recognizes that the power of love, compassion, community, and intention are as important to healing as any of our pills and medicines, and possibly more powerful...[205]

Lawlis became interested in transpersonal approaches as he worked to help patients control pain. He states that transpersonal medicine is:

> ...based on people's experience of transcending their usual identification with their limited biological, historical, cultural, and personal selves and, at the most profound levels of experience possible, recognizing or even being "something" of vast intelligence and compassion that encompasses the entire universe.... the transpersonal, which experientially impresses us with our fundamental unity with each other and all life...[206]

As Lawlis continued his research, he discovered the work of Jeanne Achterberg, who has pointed out the importance of ritual in healing processes across cultures and quotes her as saying that ritual is "the universal foundation for all transpersonal medicine".[207] Regular, repeated practice is one of the definitions of the word ritual, and part of the process that gives the necessary depth of meaning to the symbols.

Observing that the wide range of responses to pain medication among his patients seemed to have far less to do with the patient's bodyweight and health than with the patient's state of mind and community, Dr. Lawlis started to experiment with different approaches. Visualization, Progressive Relaxation, and simply listening were among the techniques he found effective, with consistently higher results in cases where groups worked together to support individuals.

This is not surprising, because all the guidelines for effective imagery start with the same instructions: relax the body and still the mind, focusing on the emerging image and letting awareness of

A New Model of the Healing Process

external events slip away. Clearly, these guidelines elicit Benson's Relaxation Response, which has been found to be so effective in encouraging a sense of wellbeing. The additional effects of the inner experience provided by the imagery session augment the overall effectiveness of this technique.

Recent studies, such as those supported by the Institute of Noetic Sciences (IONS) described earlier in this book, have gone even further than Lawlis' experience, demonstrating that not only the thoughts and beliefs of the patient, but those of the doctor and other caregivers, affect the patient's recovery.

Several hundred studies focusing on the effects of prayer—by doctors and other staff, by friends and family, and by strangers—observing several thousand patients under a variety of experimental conditions, have established that the kind of intense positive regard with an intention of well-being for the patient that we call prayer results in significant improvements in responses to medical procedures, speeds recovery from such procedures, and reduces the number and severity of side effects associated with the procedures and with hospital care.[208]

Dr. Hew Len, a Hawaian psychiatrist used an ancient Polynesian healing method called *ho'oponopono*, in a ward for the criminally insane. As described by David Wilcock in *The Source Field Investigations*.

> He simply took on their pains and problems as if they were his own, and worked on healing those issues within himself: "I just kept saying 'I'm sorry' and 'I love you' over and over again." ...Dr Len recommends going inside, to whenever you feel hurt by a particular person or issue, and then saying each of these 4 statements with as much feeling as possible—thinking through the real reasons why you genuinely feel this way: I love you; I am sorry; Please forgive me; Thank you. That's all it takes. You heal the other person be healing yourself—and this apparently works because in the greater sense, you are both sharing the same mind.[209]

Other studies, using placebos, have established a direct correlation between the caregiver's beliefs and the patient's response to the supposed treatment being offered. Among the most famous of these was the realization by a cardiologist that a common surgery for a specific heart problem did not, in fact, affect that problem, in spite of the consistently high rate of recovery for those who had gone through it.[210]

The implications of these facts for the healing process are substantial. First, it becomes necessary to recognize that the beliefs and attitudes of the care provider will affect the healing process of the patient. Beyond that, it becomes clear that whatever ideas or states are active in the collective consciousness will affect the individual—and *vice versa*—so the healer needs to be aware of the larger picture while addressing the local issue. But no aspect of the new model of the healing process is more important than the care provider's indication to the patient of the power of self-care. Specific self-care methods, such as meditation, could complete and sustain the healing.

The Power of Intention

Intention to heal oneself or others is a gift inherent in the mind-body system. In health or in illness, at any time, the energy of healing intention that one radiates into oneself or out to another person, or to several other people, really helps relieve sickness and suffering. Over 150 clinical trials have demonstrated that healing intention can be instantaneously used and directed by average people, that it is not the special gift of a few "healers." Indeed, it seems to be a gift that most or all people have and can use, which is why so many people have benefited from energy healing practices, in spite of the relatively little-known research to support its value.

> What is the energy of intention? It's something more readily experienced than explained. The energy of intention is akin to the energy of prayer, which is described as nonphysical.[211]

It's experienced not as something traveling through air or space, through which it might deteriorate, but as reaching its destination full force and instantly, in the unified field of life. This characteristic of healing intention is in accordance with our model of the body, because what shifts is the practitioner's own energy field, which instantaneously vibrates with the energy fields resonating with it across the planet. Such is our unlimited, universal nature.

The intention to heal, as Claude Swanson discovered and as Reiki and other energy practitioners learn, begins a healing process for the

A New Model of the Healing Process

practitioner as well as the receiver. Then the focus on a particular person establishes the resonant connection for the healing/healed field of the practitioner to interact with the corresponding field of the receiver, and resonates in the universal energy field. Such is the nature of resonant vibration.

Another property of the energy of healing intention is that it is integral to the light nature of the body, called the Sambhogakaya by Buddhists, and seems to work outside of normal time and space.

This suggests that the source of the power of healing intention is both our Dharmakaya, or infinite nature, and the Nirmanakaya, our manifest body.

Energy Healing Methods

Given a model of the human body that is based on energy, the inclusion of energy healing methods is essential to our model of healing. Typically, such methods as acupuncture, acupressure, reflexology, and some forms of chiropractic require extensive training for the practitioner in both diagnostic and therapeutic methods. Other energy methods, including Therapeutic Touch (also called Healing Touch), Reiki, laying on of hands, and use of crystals, are more easily learned and applied. The practitioner is trained to both diagnose the condition by "reading" the energy and treat the condition by letting energy flow through them into the patient. A practitioner may also self-administer these forms of healing. In fact, some trainers encourage students to do so as a way to practice the method. Some renowned self-care methods, including Awareness-Based Energy Breathing (p. 177) and Transformative Compassionate Breathing (p. 217), are energy healing methods.

Most energy healing methods assume our model's principle that dysfunction in the manifest body is first a dysfunction in the energy body. Self-care energy meditation can directly heal the energy body and harmonize the mind-body fields.

Energy therapy practitioners are trained to "read" the patterns in the field of energy around the body to identify potential problem areas and then they allow what we've called chi or prana, the universal life force, to flow through their own central energy channel and out through their hands to the affected energy center or physical body part.

Among Reiki practitioners (Reiki meaning "universal life energy"), it's possible to obtain additional training to learn how to "send" life force across space and time—for both diagnosis and healing. This second-degree training also provides techniques for discovering blocks in the energy channels and dissolving them. In terms of our model, of course, the only thing being "sent" is the intention—a shift in one's own energy field that resonates with the energy of the other and assists a shift there toward greater harmony and balance. Self-care energy meditation practitioners are able to align their bodies directly into greater function and harmony.

Thus we have two kinds of energy healing methods: one applied to a patient by a trained energy healing practitioner, and the other self-applied by the patient-practitioner. Practitioners of energy medicine usually prescribe empowering self-care methods to their patients and often provide training in their use,.

Among other energy healing arts that have proven to be effective are the use of needles or crystals in energy healing. They both may enhance the energy shift in the patient by either pinpointing it to specific energy channels (as in the case of acupuncture) or (in the case of crystals) a skilled doctor or healing practitioner may tune the energy of the patient to a specific frequency, helping that person regain health.

In terms of our model, the practitioner is using intention and imagery to let energy flow through them (or their needles or crystals) to restore harmony in the shared energy body of the practitioner and patient, thus facilitating a restoration of health in the patient's physical body.

The internally applied self-care energy healing methods featured in Part Three generally use intention to visualize energy and body function and so to shift into greater mind-body actualization. However effective externally applied energy therapies may be, in terms of the potential of healing, it's more empowering and enlivening to generate healing activity from within through self-care energy medicine.

> "....intuitive or symbolic sight is not a gift but a skill... a skill based in self-esteem. Developing this skill – and a healthy sense

of self – becomes easier when you can think in the words, concepts, and principals of energy medicine.[212]

The Role of Meditation

In all of the research cited in Part One of this book, one thing is perfectly clear: the practice of meditation significantly enhances the well-being of the practitioner, regardless of age or state of health when begun, and without the negative side effects of invasive, Era I medicine. In terms of the model we have developed here, we can say that the practice of meditation assists the manifest body directly through calming, and enhances the function of the energy body in two ways: by allowing the energy fields and channels to realign optimally, and by breathing vital energy into the central energy channel.

As we consider the use of meditation as a form of therapy appropriate to an Era II or Era III model of medicine, we realize that all healing depends on the kinds of results that are achieved through the practice. It is a matter of discovering which of the different forms of meditation are most appropriate for which kinds of conditions. And it is ever increasingly clear that meditation is a great preventive medicine. It can bring people to the unconditioned state.

Imagery

Although not usually considered a form of meditation in the classic Buddhist sense, many of the same characteristics apply to the use of imagery in medicine. The practice of imagery requires stopping what one is doing and focusing on an internal process, thus resting the body and ending normal thought processes.

Imagery also can be experienced as a process of alignment, harmonizing different aspects of the mind-body, in ways that are very much like what researchers have found that certain dream states provide.

As Lawlis discovered in his pain clinics, imagining being healthy or imagining an experience of becoming healthy can be very effective in reducing the discomfort of symptoms, and often the symptoms themselves.

Imagery, in all its forms, can be used to shift a patient's focus away from his or her distress, to create an alternative understanding of the situation and, through repetition, to replace old patterns of worry or fixation on the past with a new pattern of thought and feeling. This last form, commonly called "positive imagery," has been proved effective in athletics and the workplace, as well as in therapeutic settings.

Imagery is most typically used in association with chronic conditions and terminal illness. However, increasing experience with the technique proves it to be useful for reducing swelling and inflammation (decreasing pain and sinus problems), shifting blood flow from the brain to the extremities (reducing or eliminating headaches), and removing excess inches from the body (most effectively as part of a plan of diet and exercise).

Progressive Relaxation Therapies

Because of Edmund Jacobson's remarkable work demonstrating the effectiveness of progressive neuromuscular release, and through Kabat-Zinn's application of that method in his work with mindfulness meditation, we have a body of evidence and protocol for its use, and a clear understanding of the conditions that are most amenable to treatment with this method.

Indications for treatment by Progressive Relaxation include:

- acute neuromuscular hypertension
- chronic neuromuscular hypertension
- states of fatigue and exhaustion
- states of debility (convalescence from infectious and exhaustive diseases of various types)
- chronic pulmonary tuberculosis
- organic and functional heart disorders
- vascular hypertension
- preoperative and postoperative conditions
- toxic goiter
- disturbances of sleep
- alimentary spasm, including mucous colitis, colonic

spasm, cardiospasm, and esophagospasm
- peptic ulcer
- preventive medicine

Vase Breathing: Awareness-Based Energy Breathing

For centuries, breathing energy into the navel energy center has been known to be a great method for developing and maintaining optimal human function.

Vase Breathing is energy breathing meditation. It can be doubly transformative. Compared to mindfulness meditation there is a totally different sense of what breathes and what is breathed. Vase breathing is the mindful breathing of energy into the energy body. Dr. Dean Ornish has included a form of energy breathing in his plan for heart patients.

One goal of this book, given the medical potential of Vase Breathing, is to encourage research to ascertain its benefits.

Mindfulness meditation has been substantially researched, with great interest in the medical and psychological value of its benefits. Vase Breathing has the same central psychological method as mindfulness meditation but may have even more profound biological and psychological benefits because of its impact on deeper dimensions of body and breathing. We hope that research will soon support the application of Vase Breathing in medicine at least as much as it supports the application of mindfulness meditation.

Based on experience and known functionality, medical indications for the use of Vase Breathing include:

- disease prevention
- cancer care
- heart care
- HIV/AIDS care
- near-death care
- anxiety
- depression
- immune enhancement
- pain management

- complications from medication and surgery
- childbirth medicine

Transformative Compassionate Breathing

In Compassionate Breathing, the act of breathing becomes very powerful. Simply going with the natural flow of the breath, one breathes in, taking into the energy body the energy of any sickness and suffering of any living person—oneself or anyone else. The energy breathed in dissolves into light in the energy body, and then energy of healing intention is breathed out into whomever one intends to heal, wherever they are. The nonlocal nature of our mind-body means that we can merge our intention with another person and it may be felt by the person we focus on. It may also reach all others with similar patterns of energy.

A powerful illustration of this method occurred in Tibet, in the eleventh century. Leprosy was common, and ordinary doctors didn't know how to cure it. Perhaps it could be compared to AIDS today. A lama named Geshe Chekhawa taught Compassionate Breathing, called *Tong Len*, in Tibet, to a group of lepers. "Many of the lepers who did Tong Len practice were cured. The news of this spread fast, and many other lepers flocked to his house".[213]

Let's apply this in today's terms. A person suffering with leprosy or AIDS goes to a lama, a spiritual teacher, pleading for help. The teacher says to that person that there is a method that might be able to cure them. The suffering person would have to practice the method by himself or herself, and practice it intensively. They would have to be willing to drop their suffering, to forget about it, and compassionately open their heart to another suffering person, someone suffering the same disease. They practice healing others and themselves, using their inherent healing ability, rather than focusing on their own suffering. The more completely the practice is done, they're told, the more likely it will be to bring healing to the person who does the practice.

Describing compassion or *Bodhicitta* (bodhi meaning "enlightened essence" and citta meaning "heart"), Shantideva writes:

> It is the supreme elixir
>
> that overcomes the sovereignty of death.

> It is the inexhaustible treasure
> that eliminates poverty in the world.
> It is the supreme medicine
> that quells the world's disease. (ibid., 201)

When people drop their suffering self-nature and turn attention to their energy body's potential, they shift their state of consciousness from one of illness into the innate, unconditioned functioning of the Nirmanakaya, body of compassion. In this innate state it's possible to quickly dissolve the obstructions resulting from one's conditioned functioning because one is inherently free of that conditioning.

With the practice of Compassionate Breathing anyone can turn directly to their life force and enter the great potential of Dharmakaya, unlimited life, removing all obstructions to one's own health. Compassionate Breathing for oneself and others doesn't waste a breath. So it's understood that compassionate breathing is a form of meditation that may be applied to any condition involving distress or suffering. Over the past decade, it has been effectively used for childbirth labor, AIDS, rheumatoid arthritis, osteoarthritis, and cancers.

Audio-Guidance

People who are semi-comatose, such as those suffering from Alzheimer's disease, those who are in deep coma, and those who are near death require healthcare methods that cover a vast range of concerns. This is an area of healthcare for which the methods of Era I medicine are considered inappropriate by many people, among them healthcare professionals and a large portion of the general public. We see controversial and expensive medical interventions used aggressively, often without improving the quality of life of the patients—who, all too often, have been subjected to such treatment without informed consent. These are healthcare fields where new methods and approaches are crucially needed.

Toward the end of his life, Carl Jung reflected on

> ...certain astonishing observations in cases of profound [unconsciousness] after acute injuries to the brain and in severe cases of [brain] collapse. In both situations, total loss of consciousness can be accompanied by perceptions of the outside

world and vivid dream experiences. Since the cerebral cortex, the seat of consciousness, is not functioning at these times, there is as yet no explanation for such phenomena.

They may be evidence for at least a subjective persistence of the capacity for consciousness—even in a state of apparent unconsciousness.[214]

Jung's "astonishing observation" concerning the indestructible and perhaps undisturbable foundation for mental activity, which we have called "inner awareness," may have been an anticipation of the turning to meditation methods in the West. Today, countless thousands of people in Western nations are discovering the nature of the inner awareness: timeless, perhaps immortal, and experientially free of disturbance and limitation.

In considering an approach to comatose, semi-comatose, and near-death states, it's useful to note that all three situations have one vital common factor: functioning in the outer world is no longer a matter of concern to that person. For each of these human conditions, the ability to access inner awareness has become important.

Because there is diminished concern for the outer world, inner awareness is more accessible. Therefore, the approach with highest potential for effectiveness in all these conditions is one that addresses the need to access inner awareness: meditation.

The question becomes, however, how can one arrange for a demented or comatose patient to meditate? One promising solution is a prerecorded guided meditation that can be played near the patient, regardless of location, activity, or condition. Medigrace, a nonprofit organization established in 1991 to advance the use of meditation in medicine, produces such recordings, calling them "audio-guides." Healthcare providers who have used them have found them to be effective in reducing the severity of symptoms in their patients, reducing stress for caregivers, and providing a means for inner release. In some cases this may allow recovery.

Attitudinal Healing Methods

In the book *Teach Only Love*, Dr. Gerald Jampolsky, a psychiatrist, describes his movement from the limitations of his training into the infinite possibility of unconditional love and acceptance. Based on

A New Model of the Healing Process

the teachings and principles of *A Course in Miracles*, Jampolsky's book outlines his transformative journey from diagnostics and treatment through loss of faith in healing to a new understanding of the nature of the therapeutic process and his own capacity to heal.

The outcome of the journey was the formation of the Center for Attitudinal Healing, presently located in Sausalito, California—which still functions, three decades after its founding.

What Jampolsky came to understand—and embodied in his Center—was that there is neither a patient nor a therapist, but two seekers together on a journey of healing. He accepted what many therapists know but do not acknowledge in their practice: that when the therapist is ready, the patient appears—exactly the perfect patient to help the therapist complete his or her own healing process.

Beyond that, he realized that the really important function of the therapist operating in the traditional model is as Listener. It was not his expertise in pharmaceuticals, nor his demonstrated ability to apply various therapeutic models, that his patients needed. It was simply his ability to sit and focus and listen, without judgment, to what they needed to express.

So, Jampolsky made a decision. He decided to change his own attitude. He decided to let go of his persona as authoritative expert and all the judgments and assessments that went with that. He decided to focus, instead, on listening to, and loving (that is, accepting unconditionally, without attachment) his patients, and, in the process, he became a healer.[215]

Not too surprisingly, this approach is very similar to the process of pastoral counseling that has recently begun to be taught to ministers, priests, and rabbis. It works—for both the counselor and the counselee.

In terms of the model presented here, what Jampolsky did was shift from Era I, invasive medicine to Era III, transpersonal medicine. He stopped operating as if the patient were a body with emotions and started sensing the whole, complex being—including the multidimensional bodies. He started to acknowledge that he could never do just one thing, and recognized that for either participant in the healing process to experience a greater degree of wholeness was for both of them to—and he let the patient guide the process, more often than not.

When we change our attitude, we do, in fact, change the pattern of energy that we are in the world. When we free our attitude and experience fresh potential, we can raise the level of function in our body.

The Healer

As the 21st century brings greater use of Era III transpersonal medicine, ordinary people begin to recognize and use their innate ability to heal themselves and others by practicing energy meditation methods.

In this book we've spoken of faith healers, New Thought healers, and various healing arts practitioners, as acknowledging human healing potential more fully than Era I scientific medicine. Working from an incomplete model of the human mind-body system, Era I medical pracitioners assume that the patient is a passive receiver of healing modalities, primarily drugs and surgery, provided by knowledgeable physicians and their assistants. Though some physicians will go so far as to say that they are "helping the body to heal itself," recognizing the marvelous, complex systems within the body for restoring health, most are convinced that it's the tools they use that do the work.

We've explored how some non-western traditions work with an expanded model. In the shamanic traditions, for example, the patient is seen as an active participant in the healing process, along with friends and family. Healing is a process that involves body, mind, spirit, and community. Individualized protocols are developed to assist the patient through the specific combination of actions and experiences that will undo the distress and restore wellbeing for all concerned. Often these include some forms of medicine, along with some psycho-emotional experiences and, often, spiritual counseling. The healer's role is that of facilitator.

Even in faith healing and the New Thought tradition the practitioner is a facilitator: the patient must do the healing.

The energy medicine practitioner acts as a conduit of energy and a perceiver of specific blocks to energy flows, with the expectation that the patient's will and openness are what allow the energy to do its work in the body. It's understood that maintaining a healthy flow of energy to and through all parts of the body is essential for wellbeing and that the healing therapist's role is to assist the patient in re-creating such a flow. When patients are their own energy medicine practitioners, it's in shifting attention from mind to awareness that they shift back to a healthier energy flow.

Across these modalities, both the external healer and the internal healer see the person needing healing as a complex energetic system that may be influenced by thought as well as action. Will and openness can unlock blocked energy flows from the inside. This is the healthiest kind of medicine, the most empowering.

As the medical establishment lingers on the verge of collapse, and as the era of self-care-centered care is upon us, people in general will have to change their minds by means of meditation. There will be too few energy arts practitioners and true healing practitioners for the massive populations that will need healthcare. Era III medicine, therefore, is universal medicine, and anyone can and should be a healer.

An Integrated Model of the Healing Process

More and more, the evidence tells us that the healing process is fundamentally a change of mind. In *When the Body Says No*, Gabor Maté tells us that

> Whichever modality of treatment people choose— conventional medicine with or without complementary healing alternative approaches like energy medicine or various mind-body techniques; ancient Eastern practices like Ayurvedic medicine or various mind-body techniques; the universal practice of meditation techniques; psychotherapy; nutritional healing... There are many different ways to find that innate capacity for freedom, outlined in many teachings... [healing] is only possible if we first liberate ourselves from the tyranny of our ingrained biology of belief.[216]

Healing is not only bringing the body back to normal function. As it liberates the mind the healing process may bring the whole person to greater than normal function.

This means that, as we consider each of these healing approaches in light of the model of the human body that we've offered, we can explain the role they play in bringing about a new, more fully functional state of being.

In the context of our model of the body as interacting fields of resonant energy manifesting in a material form, we can see that the meditation practices of Progressive Relaxation and Vase Breathing permit the individual to rest in the innate harmony of the multidimensional body. They thereby restoring that harmony and balance within the energy body and the physical body that it manifests. The energy associated with prayer, positive imagery, and listening with love has the effect of restoring a harmonious energy pattern where there has been dysfunction.

One element of our model is that dysfunction occurs first in the energy body, either through misaligned fields or through blocked energy channels. Clearly, energy healing methods are useful for treating these conditions—methods either self-administered or provided by a trained practitioner. In addition, the meditation technique of Vase Breathing is specifically designed to restore harmony and balance to the fields and structures of the energy body.

Another element in our model is the transpersonal nature of the mind-body system. Being continually in interaction with all other beings on the planet, we need healing methods that honor those connections and help us to utilize them effectively. The methods of prayer, distance Reiki, and Compassionate Breathing all honor the transpersonal nature of our being and give us means for shifting our attention from our own concerns to the concerns of others and their healing, while simultaneously drawing into our energy body the necessary energy for healing ourselves.

Finally, our model states that we are fundamentally not material bodies, but energetic wave-forms that function outside of the normal 3-dimensional material reality. As energy, we're not limited by the location of our material bodies and can function anywhere in the universe at any time. This means we have the potential for operating not only everywhere on this planet at any instant, but all the processes and experiences of the whole space-time continuum are available to everyone. So, in the depths of the awareness of the energetic human body is all-knowing primordial awareness, perfect sanity, perfect health. And we can all access it any time we "turn off" our normal, matter-bound thought processes.

A New Model of the Healing Process 151

Our model says that the material body is dependent on a continuous flow of energy for its wellbeing. When the energy body is out of alignment, the flow of universal energy through our matieral body systems is impaired and the systems may dissipate as a result. If the human body has dissipated to the point where consciousness is no longer identified with it, healing may come in the form of audio-guidance into the next stage of life—generally called death. When there is still life, Era II and III energy body methods have the capacity to restore function—even when drugs, surgery, and other treatments have failed. The best use of such methods, however, is to maintain health and prevent disorder.

Our model states clearly that, for greater functioning, greater life, the best interventions are those which support enhanced energy flows in the body and minimize interruptions of those flows. The methods presented in Part Three are a step into the potential of this Era III medicine for restoring health and wellbeing in all circumstances and for all conditions.

PART THREE: METHODS FOR SELF-CARE AND FOR THE HEALING OF OTHERS

A new model of the mind-body and a new paradigm for the healing process suggest new methods and explain the effectiveness of old ones. In this next section we offer versions of several ancient methods for healing self and others that have been demonstrated to work as transformative, as well as healing, processes.

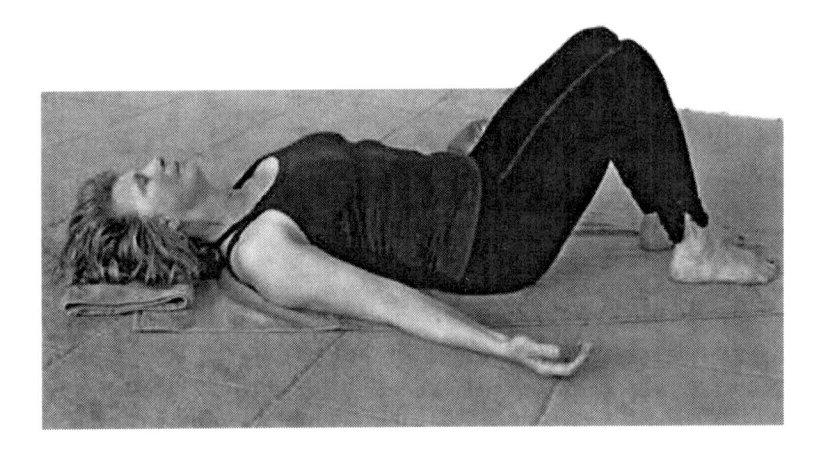

Deep Release: one body position that can work
for progressive relaxation.

Deep Release

Before any mind-body method can be effective, the body must be relaxed and comfortable. Relaxation is often, therefore, an element of techniques such as meditation, hypnosis, and yoga. Nonetheless, there is one relaxation technique that stands out and has been extensively studied: progressive muscle relaxation. It was originally developed by Edmund Jacobson and presented to the public in 1938 as a technique requiring dozens of sessions wherein the subject was taught to relax approximately thirty different muscle groups.[217] Using this approach, Jacobson helped people heal nervous system conditions corresponding to a wide range of disorders.

Dr. Jacobson developed many Progressive Relaxation (PR) techniques throughout a distinguished clinical and research career at the Harvard Medical School and then at the University of Chicago Medical School, from the 1930s through the 1940s. They ranged from isometric exercises for specific muscle groups to total system methods. The object of all the methods was to release muscular stresses on the nervous system in order to treat nervous system impacts on health.

> Because of reflex connections, the nervous system cannot be quieted except in conjunction with the muscular system... The neuromuscular factor as a cause and element of the symptomatology of various disease processes has seemed evident.[218]

Quieting the nerves through muscle group relaxation he was able to treat the nervous system and reverse conditions it caused.

> Relaxation evidently applies to a larger field of disorders, since various conditions in internal medicine which are not psychogenic come within its scope.[219]

Nervous hypertension with fatigability ("neurasthenia") is a widespread condition, characterized by nervous tension and various associated disorders, often causing the inability to sit still. Jacobson's isometric and whole-body relaxation procedures helped the mind-body calm down therapeutically. Some of his methods were sitting practices, many were reclining, but they all made people stop and alter their function by themselves.

In the treatment of nervous states, there is increasing evidence that the subsidence of symptoms becomes most marked upon the disappearance of residual [muscular] tensions.[220]

This kind of healing work done by patients as a direct and effective way of treating many disease conditions was the first practice of self-care medicine. The location of the work was The Harvard Medical School, where the science of mind-body medicine would be developed, by Walter Cannon, MD, in the 1940s and 1950s, and by Herbert Benson, MD, from the late 1960s to the present.

Integral to Jacobson's work was Sir William Osler's knowledge of the use of rest in medicine. Rest and self-care, shifting responsibility to the patient, were the basis of a breakthrough in therapeutic direction. The emphasis in treatment programs shifted from care in the medical office to home care.

> The aim of nervous system treatment will be to point out to the patient the voluntary element in these symptoms and to guide him to rid himself of them.[221]

When Jacobson imparted his methods to his patients, he made it clear that it was essential that the patients needed to apply the methods regularly at home as self-care. In fact, Jacobson was the first published medical practitioner developing methods in which self-care would be emphasized. He anticipated the potential for self-care in a new era of medicine. Dr. Jacobson quietly initiated the new paradigm and gave it effective methods.

Jacobson's system was simplified by Douglas Bernstein and Thomas Borovec,[222] and since then, other professionals have modified his methods even further. In 1979 Jon Kabat-Zinn introduced Jacobson's full-body PR in a 45-minute "body scan" integral to the groundbreaking program at UMMC.[223] There, a new dimension was added to Jacobson's method, making it more efficient and even more effective: mindfulness meditation.

The Method

Integrating the time-honored method of mindfulness meditation, a method by which people are able to control attention and maintain focus in spite of the disturbances of the mind, made PR more effective than ever. Instead of being limited by disturbances of the

Deep Release

mind, the practice becomes awareness-enhanced, treating the mind and the nerves. And, as we explored earlier in this text, patients and doctors have identified multiple benefits of mindfulness meditation with PR.

In 1997 MediGrace, a nonprofit corporation established to extend the use of meditation in medicine, further developed mindfulness-based PR, to give it even greater potential in both preventing and reversing disease conditions. The essential features added by MediGrace are:

- Instructions to receive life force on a cellular level
- instructions to experience light in the cells and the nerves.
- rest in a new state of consciousness, free of conditions

Since 1997 MediGrace[224] has used what we call "Practice of Deep Release" in more than 100 hospital trainings. More than 12,000 people have used the method in their self-care.

The practice that follows is a version of the instruction offered in the MediGrace audio-guide #MG3, entitled *Calm Healing*. Like meditation, this reclining self-care practice is potentially powerful, dependent upon regular use.

Introduction

This practice is for anyone who needs energy and healing.

It's done lying down.

It's really good for nervousness and stress.

It's good for pain management and improved function.

It's good for a new sense of vital body.

In this practice you slowly go through your whole body and relax it, patiently.

You save energy and you gain new energy, new resource.

The energy increase is essential for healing and it brings calm.

It will take about twenty-five minutes to go through the process.

Find yourself a comfortable place to lie down.

If you're bedridden, lie flat on your back and straighten your body if you can.

If you're able to lie down on the floor, a mat or blankets or a rug is ideal for doing this practice.

The effects are immediate and they also build up over time.

The most benefits come from doing it every day.

It's a direct way of relaxing into energy and healing.

Make sure that you're going to be warm enough, and lie down mindfully.

Be aware that you're not lying down to take a nap and avoid falling asleep.

Keep your eyes open and softly focused.

You may close your eyes briefly from time to time to rest them and to see into life inside, but keep your eyes open as much as possible to keep from falling asleep.

If you stay awake and alert you'll find new energy fields; new potential.

As much as you do the practice, you come into your potential more and more.

Be patient with this practice.

Be patient with yourself.

Especially if you're suffering a chronic condition with physical or mental pain, do this practice again and again, to relax the tensions caused by the pain, to open to something new.

Stay in your living presence.

This practice is designed to make you confident, energized, and calm.

The energy works directly to make you well.

The Practice

> When you're ready, take a deep breath and then exhale easily.
>
> Begin feeling the sensation of life energy working in all your body at once.
>
> Take another deep breath,

deep into life,

and breathe out the release your systems need for improved function.

As if you're doing it for the first time,

come into your whole body at once.

Feel the trillions of living cells and energy flows.

Let yourself feel all the sensations of having a live human body.

There's so much life in it, it's inconceivable—

ten trillion living cells, all working together with the force of life in you.

When you feel your whole body directly,

it feels like unlimited life.

Keep feeling the sensation of all your life currents

and your electromagnetic body form.

Feel all the life going on in you at once.

Feel the cohesion.

As you become aware of life itself in you, just relax into that.

Let go of pain,

again and again and again.

Let go of suffering again and again.

Let go of any tensions or constrictions.

You're going to take this time to relax yourself all the way through,

slowly but surely.

Soon you'll feel more and more of your body,

feeling more of all the life in it at once.

You go through your body,
from your feet to your head,
to take muscle pressure off your nerves.

For the sake of your nerves
you need to release unconscious tension in your muscle systems.

Stay in touch with the sensation of life in your whole body,
from the crown down.
Starting with the toes of your left foot,
feel all the life in your toes.

Feel the functions of the bones—
all that they always do that you don't notice.

Feel the channels of energy that run through your feet.

Feel how it all works together.
Feel your toes and all of your foot vibrating together.

Feel how much life there is in it.

If there is any tension or pain,
locate exactly where,
and relax the muscles and tendons there.

Let them open into the total current.

Feel in your foot all the work it has been doing for your body all these years.

Relax any clenched muscles or tension in your tendons.

Open whatever needs to be opened.
Relax it into its open-and-ready state.

There may be muscles and tendons that haven't relaxed for years.
You are there inside them, so just let them open.

Feel how this benefits your arteries and your nerves.

Bring your attention from your left foot into your left ankle.
Feel all the energy flows going through it, to and from all parts of your body.

Find and relax any tight muscle or tendon.
Let your ankle relax into its softness, pliant and able.

Feel the goodness of the electrical flow,

the goodness of the blood flow,

and the connection with all the life flows in your body.

Know them now.

Let your awareness move up into the calf of your left leg.

Feel all the muscles in your calf.

Be aware of all the work these muscles do in helping you maintain your life.

Appreciate that.

Have a good feeling for what is there, and then relax it.

Let it open.

Let your flesh and bone feel its aliveness.

All throughout your foot and lower leg,

feel, relax, and open all the muscles you can find.

Find them all.

Relax them all.

Relax anything that feels like tension in the nerves of your lower leg.

Feel healed and whole throughout your lower leg and foot.

Now go up through your left knee.

Feel all the sensation in your knee.

This is a good way to meditate, going through your body,

knowing your body as if for the first time.

Let your body save energy and heal by opening and coming alive.

Come up into your left thigh.
Feel how your thigh supports your body in life.

Feel its energy. Release any tension that's there.

Effortlessly relax all you can throughout your entire left leg.
There may be tensions there that have been tight for years.
Just find them. You're there inside them.

All throughout your leg and foot feel the big muscles and the small ones.
Feel it all together. And relax it all together.

Feel a relaxing and healing in your nerves.

Feel your blood flow with all the wonderful work it does.

Feel all your life flow sensation.

Open into it all.

Rest into it all.

Now notice your right foot.
Feel the toes of the foot.

Feel all the life in each toe.

Continue to feel your whole left leg.

The life current of that is with you as you go through your right leg.

Everything you've brought your attention to is still in your awareness

as you go through more and more of your body,

releasing tensions and increasing function.

You unlock blocked systems, taking care of your own needs,

taking out the basis of any harmful condition,

coming to the basis of new life.

In your right foot, contact all the bones and the life-fields.

Through the ball of your foot and the arch,

feel all the work your foot does for you.

Feel all the life service in your foot.

On its sensitive sole,

feel the bottom of your energy body.

Let go of old patterns affecting your nervous system,

releasing your nerves for new function.

Come up through your right ankle, relaxing it.

Moving upwards, sense your body fields.

Come up into the calf of your right leg,
feeling the vibrations of its flesh and bone.

Find and open all the muscles in your calf,
releasing any constricted flows.
Heal into your energy fields.

Open more of anything needing to be relaxed in your legs.
Release more and more of any tensions limiting the full flow of life,
in the flesh and in the bone.

Feel more of the sensation of life in your flesh.

Relax whatever may be habitually tense.
Feel the energy gain when you relax.

Come up from your right calf through the sensation in your knee, into your thigh.
In an enlivening way you're coming through more and more of your body.

You have unused resource to heal into.
To heal into it you have to let go.

The sensation of all the life in us at once is available all the time,
but unless you give it attention you live without its benefits.

Becoming still and letting go,

we heal into deep body sensation.

It's the body of life free of all conditioning,

the basis of wholeness and healing.

Now, in both your legs,

throughout all the muscles and tendons,

blood vessels and nerves,

there's a growing sense of ease.

If any pain or tension persists in you,

breathe into and out of the pain and tension.

Feel how muscles tighten all around pain in resistance,

trying to block it out.

Relax the muscle clench

and accommodate the pain or tension.

Breathe it in and give it space.

The key is not to identify with the pain.

Breathe into and out of that area if you need to at any time,

but keep with the direction of this practice,

continuing to enter unused resource.

Relax more and more,

in greater awareness,

with your nerves working in a more healed way.

Come from your thighs up through your loins into your belly:

your navel and solar plexus power centers.

Feel the whole lower half of your body,

from your abdomen down.

Feel all the life and life support in it.

Now once again, feel your whole body,

deeper and more completely.

Feel the dynamics of your central nervous system,

taking care of billions of functions at once.

Feel the energy of all your higher systems,

silently performing countless activities,

ingeniously working,

ceaselessly working for greater life.

Feel that you embody the realization of life.

You were born to have and experience this all.

It's time to be what you really are:

a body inconceivably alive.

Breathe into any areas of tension or pain.
Welcome the electronic sensations,
to come into the greater life you have.

Staying relaxed in your abdomen and breathing there,
see wonderful living systems in yourself.

Since they are yours, you can know them,
and enter the bliss of all the life at work in you,
life giving you pulsing potential.

Sense other-dimensional bodies in your cells.

See the light of all your electromagnetic flows.

Heal your pains into the unity of that light.

Now in your abdomen and your solar plexus
feel any tensions collected there over the years.

Stay in your navel, breathing easily and deeply.
You are there, inside, and now your attention is in there too.
You know your own gut area.
Open more of all the holding, all the resisting.

Let go more and more of the results of your habitual actions and your impending actions.
Relax it all.

Deep Release

Free yourself completely from actions.
Free yourself from the stress and activity of life.

Free yourself from the built-up tensions of your lifetime.
Free yourself to relax into your being, your unconditioned life.

In stillness, and in peace, heal into it.

Relax every small and large muscle in your belly and solar plexus.
Feel how that enhances the relaxing of your nerves for greater function.

Come up into your upper body.
Relax all the musculature throughout your chest.

Find any muscles contracted or partly contracted throughout your rib cage,
and around your ribs.
Feel any collected tension in your chest.

Release all tension from within.
You can do it now.

Spontaneously relax it all from within.

Open your chest and shoulders,
breathing in deeply,

and relax as you exhale and release.

Come into your heart..

Enter the dynamic majesty of your heartwork.

Be thankful that it runs itself so well.

Appreciate its power, and how every cell in your body helps it beat.

Be all the light of the electricity in its beats.

Feel the gift of miracles within miracles making all this life flow, with force.

See that the powerful blood beat is full of your light.

See your body-light in all your systems.

Feel with the full force of your embodiment that you are healing in all this life.

The very presence of all this life in you is your healing.

Now feel your whole back.

Feel whatever tensions there may be in the spine.

Where gravity and personal tensions have been compressing or fusing vertebrae,

let that stop.

Let the bone spontaneously unlock.

Let your whole spine open.

Feel its bones and nerves adjust, ready to realign.

Come up your spine, through your shoulders,
and into your neck.
Open, and let sensation flow.

The tension of daily living can tense the head and spine.
Spontaneously relax it all from within.
It could seem difficult, but simply unlock the built-up tensions
of your upper body and neck.

Feel the natural ease of releasing any contraction
in your back and neck and head.

Let the muscles loosen.
Feel the energy gain.

Let it flow, enlivening you..

Relax all the muscles around your head,
muscles connecting your head to your neck and shoulders.
Relax in the awareness that comes alive when important life
energy is gained.

From head to toe,

feel the cohesion of coming together in total flow of life sensation.

If you want to flow free instead of wasting energy in unconscious tensions,

feel how natural it is to be at ease in deep release.

Check your head and neck for any remaining tension.

Save energy, letting any holding unfold.

Let it all melt down.

Time to let it all be naturally soft.

Let the fields in your body come into union.

Come into your face now, starting with your jaw.

Breathe into it and let your jaw loosen,

completely letting go of the need to speak.

All throughout your lower face, feel any muscular tension, and relax it.

Give your jaw a chance to really rest,

to save your energy, and your teeth.

Start reversing any tension in your mouth.

Let it be in its natural ease.

Feel all the different sets of muscles in your mouth,

forming your expressions, conscious and unconscious.

Find all those muscles, and relax them.

Release all the residual expression and the tendency to expression.

Let your mouth be free of that now.

Relax into a state where you are free of active tendencies,

free in unconditioned body,

free in unconditioned life.

Relax your jaw,

your mouth,

and your cheeks.

Relax your entire lower face

into the total sensation of life energy.

Feel all habitual patterns dissolving in greater awareness.

Now feel all the muscles connected to your eyes,

forming the expression in and around them,

habitual and spontaneous expression, all that you know as yourself.

Move carefully through your eye muscles,

relaxing that musculature, more and more.

Move carefully through the muscles around your right eye.

Relax any tension you find.

Now go through the muscles around your left eye, relaxing them.

Release the potential of expression around both your eyes.

Let your eyes rest in themselves.

Feeling yourself becoming free,
relax into the free body of life you are.

Rest free of all external activity now,
and free of conscious and unconscious mind.

Rest free of any harmful conditioning in your body channels.

Feel like you're coming alive for the first time.

Rest in freedom from life and death.

From your eyes come up into your brows and forehead.
Feel your forehead muscles latent with expressions.
Now, consciously, throughout your forehead,
relax any overt or subtle expression.
Relax into your inherent open awareness,
free of life and death.

Now feel both your arms at once, flowing with life.

Feel all the life expression in your arms and hands.
Feel the life energies in the fingers of both hands.

Feel life force throughout your fingers and hands.

Feel the inherent healing capability in your hands.

Feel all the vital channels in your wrists.

Relax any subtle tensions in your hands and wrists.

More and more,
feel the bliss of normal function in your body,
as if coming into it with awareness for the first time.

Feel your forearms
and come up through your elbows
into your upper arms.
Feel the activity potential of your arms and hands.
Feel the blessing and goodness of that.

Feel all of both arms at once,
relaxing all the tendencies into the activities of life
to come into inner resource.

Relax in inaction.
Connect with inner awareness.

Free yourself from the actions of body, speech, and mind.
Enter the deathless energy of greater awareness.

And now again,
sense your multidimensional body of life, all at once.

Be more in contact than you've ever been with your greater life.

Heal into that greater life.

Come to it more and more.

Sense that it is unlimited.
It is your unlimited potential.
Use this practice to come to life, again and again, to feel well.

Open your muscle and nerve body into your energy body every day.
Let yourself feel the healing and life energy gain.

The more you give to the practice,

the more you heal.

Feeling more and more at ease in deep release

feel all your systems flowing with life.

Resting in inaction

you come in a fresh way to your potential.

Follow this procedure. Again and again come through your whole body, to rest free of the basis of any harmful conditions.

In ending this practice, break stillness with awareness. See how much you can be aware of timelessness as you move.

Awareness-Based Energy Breathing

In several of the master paths developed in human history, breathing vital energy into the navel energy center is the heart of the practice.

In Tai Chi, one is directed to "sink the chi into the dantien," meaning breathe chi in and down into the energy body, into an energy form in the navel center that receives and stores chi. It's said to be located about 3 finger widths below and two finger widths behind the navel. The dantien is the physical center of gravity in the human body.

In Zen meditation, people breathe into the tanden, also called Hara, "vital center", behind and just below the center of the navel. Masters of various arts, including calligraphy, swordsmanship, tea ceremony, and martial arts, among others, are said to be "acting from the hara" when they perform masterfully.

In the Hindu yoga tradition the navel chakra in the energy body, swadhisthana, is known as the seat of prana, radiating out into the whole body. Breathing vital energy in the air down into the navel energy center is called pranic breathing.

In Buddhist Vajrayana meditation, one breathes prana into the Life Vase, tse bum (Tibetan), the Vase of Immortality, in the energy body centered behind the navel, between four finger widths above and four finger widths below, where the womb is in women.[225] *Tse* is one of several words for life in Tibetan; *bum* means vase. Both men and women are made to breathe into their inherent life vase. Breathing life-giving energy of the universal field into the *tse bum* is called vase breathing. It is complete breathing.

In all traditions the benefits of breathing energy into the energy body have been cited as increased vitality and longevity. With respect to healthcare today, looking at the potential biological and psychological benefits of awareness-based energy breathing, as stated earlier research should increasingly reveal that this kind of meditation has the same benefits as mindfulness meditation, with additional health benefits resulting from the breathing of vital energy.

The Method

Vase breathing, *bum chung,* is awareness-based energy breathing. The practice is directly related to the tummo heat yoga meditation excitedly observed by Harvard research teams under the direction of Herbert Benson.[226] The practice Benson observed is bum chen, "big vase breathing", which is like kundalini yoga and can be dangerous to the nervous system.[227]

Bum chung, "small vase breathing", has been used in healthcare practice since 1997 by Medigrace. It has been used in hospital trainings for cancer care, heart care, pain and anxiety management, and childbirth.

In this form of meditation, breathwork is transformative. When you breathe energy you are your energy body. The focus of the practice is on the natural, uncontrived movement of breathing through which energy flows into the energy body. Awareness of and identification with breathing is the calming basis of the return to fundamental awareness, the basis of the shift out of the disorder of mind.

Staying with the breath, no matter how the mind tries to take your attention, is transformative in itself. In the Vase Breathing practice, awareness becomes energy breathing, and in sustained, conscious energy breathing is the power to transform, heal, and evolve.

In mindfulness meditation, body is ordinary and breathing is ordinary—profound but ordinary. In many therapeutic methods, breathing with the belly and centering awareness there are important as a practical discipline. In Vase Breathing, the body is extraordinary and breathing is extraordinary. There is a radically different sense of the body and its breathing capability, plus a radically different sense of air and the field of life.

In ordinary deep breathing, which is certainly healthy, air is understood to be the source of oxygen vital for life. In Vase Breathing one breathes more completely, breathing oxygen and energy, breathing with the energy body and the physical body at once. There is an experience of functioning more completely. It is also a practice of direct return to inner awareness, free of body and mind. Vase Breathing is a dual means of healing.

The more one shifts from mind into awareness, the more one realizes the radiant nature of rigpa, awareness itself, the inner luminosity, free of obstruction; the more one experiences the nature of awareness, the more one is able to release any mind-body disorders. With Vase Breathing we simultaneously breathe vital energy into the energy body for greater function while resting in the inner light of awaremess.

Vase breathing is a visualization practice in which you imagine your energy body. The central energy channel (CEC) arises from the bottom of the life vase in the navel center. We see that we're made to breathe with our physical and energy body at once, in harmony. We're made to breathe completely to live more completely. The perennial wisdom is that we are born with a capacity to breathe energies vital to our realization of life and greater health.

In Vase Breathing, we use imagery and intention to move energy from the air down into the Vase, from which it is drawn up into the CEC, to harmonize or "balance" the operation of the subtle energy power centers, bringing higher systems to life.

How do we breathe this powerful subtle energy? First it's important to sense it in the air. Some people can see it but everyone can sense it. We've been breathing it in and out all our lives without using it. Now we breathe it in and intend that energy down. Breathe it in intentionally and send it down, into a receptive energy form. When you do you'll feel it go into the vase. You'll feel your body and function expand.

Recognizing that we've been breathing subtle energy in and out since birth without using it, we begin to sense and intentionally absorb it. By intending the life-giving universal energy into the navel breathing vase, our intention directs the chi into the energy-receiving vase.

By cultivating our inherent ability to sense and absorb the subtle energy in the air, we learn to strengthen the life force behind our immune system.

The energy is absorbed into the vase directly from the air in the lungs. It doesn't need to go into and through the blood to enter the body's systems. It is absorbed directly into the remarkable energy vase form in the navel center. From there it moves up through the central energy channel to enter and enrich every aspect of the mind-body system. And because vase breathing is a practice of optimizing the functions of the radiant energy body, it is a perfect practice to realize the luminous healing nature of awareness. It offers the experience of body and awareness as light.

This sitting meditation supports a fivefold energy gain:

1. By sitting and calming down, people save energy that would have been lost in general activity. People relax, breathe deep, and gather themselves.

2. Meditation is better than sleep for restoring energy reserves. "Numerous research projects have demonstrated that meditation is psychologically and physiologically more refreshing and energy restoring than sleep." [228]

3. People save energy that would have been lost in the ceaseless activity of the mind. By shifting from mind to awareness, people reduce or stop burning up energy in the mind. Every shift people make from mind back to awareness saves energy. It's an inherent relaxation response. Not reacting to the mind saves energy and prevents disturbance.

4. People generally breathe with inefficient, high chest, or intercostal respiration, which burns up as much as seven times more energy than deep breathing. Vase Breathing saves people from wasting energy in the wrong breathing.

5. The ability to build energy reserves directly by breathing vital energy from the air gives human beings the ability to breathe into greater health and ability.

The direct breathing of life-giving energy is more than medicine. People who breathe energy into their energy bodies experience greater vitality and well-being. This may be an effective treatment for most disease conditions and for some psychophysical problems. It is also strong preventive medicine.

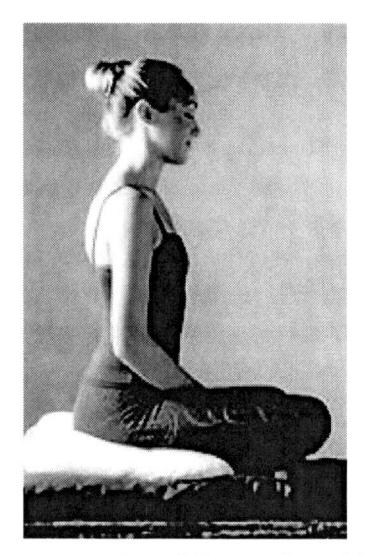

Awareness-based Energy Breathing:
the ideal body position for all forms of
mindfulness meditation.

Important: Vase Breathing is an effortless practice. There's no manipulation of the breath, no regulation. It's natural deep breathing the body likes to do. The more you do the practice consciously, the more you find yourself doing it unconsciously, letting your breathing slow down and deepen on its own. Whether your in-breath is small or is larger at any moment doesn't matter. What matters is that you are effortlessly and naturally breathing energy and oxygen at once, and you can feel how your body likes breathing completely.

On the exhale, just breathe out a little slower than you breathe in, lightly retaining the energy you breathe in. It's a gently controlled release that becomes effortless.

Introduction

You sit and visualize the radiant energetic activity of your body, with your brilliant chakra power centers and other energy body features. You see that you have a breathing vase in your navel center, an energy form made to breathe life-giving energy from the air. You sense that you were made to breathe vital energy from the air.

You use your double breathing intelligence. You breathe with your two bodies at once. You breathe energy medicine in the air and oxygen. What breathes is a deep-breathing body of awareness.

In the beginning, do this sitting practice for fifteen or twenty minutes each time. And do the practice at least once a day. If possible use cushions and sit on the floor. If you have pain or discomfort, sit in a chair with your spine balanced upright. If you're bedridden, cushions or pillows can help you raise your back as upright as possible. It's not the spine so much as the central energy channel that's being held upright, to help you to greater awareness and greater function.

The Practice

Sit into your body as if you're sitting to come to life.

Sit into your body as if you're sitting into life itself.

Sit upright, relax, and let yourself be still.

Feel the sensation of all the life in you at once.

Feel the aliveness in the stillness.

Adjust your body a little if you need to.

You should be relaxed and alert,

feeling stable and balanced.

See how that helps you feel well.

Keep coming back to the sensation

of all the energy currents moving in your body at once.

See how that feels like a direct experience of healing.

By being quiet and calming down

you come into unlimited life.

It's always there in you..

Every moment you come back to it
is a moment of instant healing.

You're going to breathe in a new way.

Both the way you breathe and what you breathe
will be extraordinary, but completely natural.
You won't be forcing your breathing at all.

Breathe with your belly.
Practice natural abdominal breathing, easy and deep.

Imagine that your whole nervous system and all your
energy channels are full of light.
And inside your navel area
is a luminous vase made of energy.
It's there to help you breathe completely.

So we sit and keep the vision of our body being full of light
and having a special breathing purpose.

Maybe for the first time in our lives
we breathe life-giving energy in the air,
something that's always been there.
We've just never related to it.
Now we see that by relating to vital energy in the air,

by breathing it in intentionally,

that energy absorbs into the vase and into our central energy channel.

Now we see that not only do we have a special breathing vase

for healing the life force,

but the medicine energies we need for healing

are in the air we've been breathing.

We've always breathed them in and out without absorbing them.

Now we're going to feed on those energies

as if they've been given to us as the perfect medicine we need,

to heal into greater health and wisdom.

Get the feeling that the vital essence you need is in the air,

and you're born to breathe it,

to live on that essence.

Do it.

See that there's fine food matter in the air

and you were born to feed on it.

Breathe energy from the air into your Vase.

Please do it now………………………………………

So we're just going to sit,

as upright as possible,

comfortable and at ease,

and practice breathing vital energies

with the Vase in our bellies.

And as you do it,

without knowing what happens,

your mind may take you out. You lose awareness..

In an instant you're lost in thought.

We're no longer breathing medicine energies,

you're thinking.

You're thinking about something,

something that happened

or something that's going to happen.

You're possibly anxious about something behind the thought.

You're not present.

You're thinking and not aware of your presence.

Then something in you that wants to live wakes up.

Awareness in you that wants to be present,

awareness that wants to be breathing vital energies,

snaps you out of the trance of thinking and wakes you up.

You come back to presence.

Keep breathing vital energy with the Vase in your belly……………………………

See how your mind takes you away from that,

then see how you wake up,

come to,

come back to the Vase Breathing.

Please do it………………………………………………………………………..

Be patient.
Be persevering to breathe in this deeper way,
this healthier way.
It helps calm you down.
It helps quiet your nerves.

If you breathe this way
You won't waste precious energy on your thinking mind.

Don't identify with your thinking mind at all as it tries to take you out.

Stay with your Vase Breathing in open awareness.

You save the energy you'd be losing in your mind
and you take in new energy from the air you breathe.

You breathe essential energy down into the Vase,
naturally and easily,
with your abdominal muscles relaxed.
The finer matter from the air absorbs into your higher systems.

See how you save vital energy and take in vital energy
by not reacting to mind as it speaks and thinks.
Calm down into your body. Breathe completely.

Please do it. Breathe free………………………..

Fears may arise,

in different ways,

causing anxious thoughts.

It is very important to recognize those thoughts,

those fears.

They may distract you from being present.

It's important to recognize anxiety. It will keep coming up.

Let it be.

Let go of it

and return to the deep breathing.

You'll see that you can do that.

If you recognize what happens in your mind and don't identify with it,

if you see it and free it, you'll feel freer,

healthier, better.

Please do it. Breathe energy from the air into the Vase……………………………..

If you catch yourself being conscious of looking at something,

or hearing something,

just recognize that you were getting lost in that.

Expand your awareness.

Sense the light of your awareness.

Return to deep breathing.

Whatever comes up—

thought,

perception,

emotion—

let it come up..

See it and free it.

Calm down into your awareness.

More and more,

understand your natural ability to be free of your mind,

to be in your body in a more healed way.

Breathe free……………………………………………………………..

Feel that the energy you absorb in the vase

may be all you need to heal with.

If you breathe this way and don't identify with what comes up in your mind,

you'll come into new function, greater function.

Please do it………………………………………………………………..

Catch the thought as it comes up
and let it be free.

Don't attach to it.

Don't fix on it.

Stay in your open awareness free of your mind.
Stay with the Vase Breathing.
Do it day and night.
Do it to heal in your sleep.

Calm down to where you are present as thought happens, as it comes up.

Leave it alone.
It changes.

It doesn't matter what the thinking is,
let it change,
and dissolve.

Stay calm.
Don't be disturbed by or taken out by your thought.
Don't be disturbed by emotions that come up.

Stay with Vase Breathing and open awareness,
and you can be undisturbable when your fears come up.

You can be undisturbable even when death comes.

Stay with the total sensation of your body.

Feel your awareness become more alive.

Sit into life beyond life and death.
Please do it……………………………………………………………….

So train yourself in this way.
Train to use the ability you have
to stay out of the trances of your mind.
Stay in the live presence of your open awareness.

Sense all of the universe, all of life, present here and now.

Sense how you can come directly to life.

Just keep to the Vase Breathing and open awareness.

Stay free of mind.

Come into presence more and more.
Breathe into presence more and more.

If you have persistent pain,

breathe into and out of the pain sensations.

Relax the region of the pain more and more.

Don't let your mind make a big deal about the pain.

Breathe into it and breathe it out more and more.

See how much energy you save by coming to the pain and staying with it.

You can prevent your own suffering.

Feel the pain out.

Feel the constrictions,

the resistance in the muscles around the pain.

Relax it intentionally more and more.

Breathe it in, and breathe it out,

until the pain eases,

as its sensations change,

and you can return to the Vase belly breathing again.

See how you save energy by working on pain directly.

When you sit into energy body,

pain sensations will change.

They may quiet down or go away.

Keep coming back to the Vase Breathing, all the time.

Please do it………………………………………………………………..

Keep shifting into open awareness.
Sense the light of awareness.

This is mind-body medicine,
and it's effective because you find it in yourself,
and in the air so vital to your life.

This is a double medicine.

Your awareness becomes medicine
when you do such practices to improve your life quality,
and the vital energy you breathe is great medicine.

Breathe it well………………………………………….

When you come to the end of this session,
as you break stillness, do it with awareness.

You're more alive.
You've done something for your health and your life.

Let yourself do it more…

Now allow your awareness to return to this time and this place and feel the energy in your body as you begin to move around and go on with your day…

Guided Imagery

The practice of guided imagery is as old as the first telling of the first story about something that happened "far away in another place." We're encouraged to relax our normal awareness and see and feel, with the narrator, the sights and sounds and textures and emotions of the time and place being described.

When Carl Simonton introduced the use of guided imagery to his patients, he really had no idea what the result would be, other than they would feel they had something to do besides sit and wait to die. What he discovered was that the simple process of imagining something was happening in their bodies actually led to measurable changes—and that was worth paying attention to.

Michael Murphy tells us "Placebo effects and spiritual healing, too, depend on suggestive imagery,"[229]

The two best known resources for guided imagery were both produced in the 1970s: Shakti Gawain's *Creative Visualization* and Jean Houston and Robert Master's *Mind Games*. Many other books include ideas and even scripts for specific imagery processes, but these two are actually texts that not only provide opportunities, but enhance one's abilities in the process.

As was discussed in Part One of this book, guided imagery has been found to be an effective healing modality. It can help reduce a variety of symptoms and has been known to turn around progressive disorders. It has also been used to reverse the accumulation of calcium in various parts of the body and to restore organ function.

Here, we shall explore one form of guided imagery, useful for general wellbeing. Later, you may wish to apply other forms of imagery for specific issues. Some specific images whose effectiveness have been demonstrated include:

- Extending a feeling of warmth to the hands and feet, from the center of the body or from an imagined stove or campfire—to reduce blood pressure or migraine pain;

- Imagining that white blood cells are white knights or little bulldozers or "pac-man" consuming a growth—to reduce the size of tumors or cysts;
- Imagining the fluid of the lymph system as slowly dissolving the build up of calcium deposits;
- Imagining the full function of a damaged organ or tissue;
- Imagining being fully active in a favorite sport;

If you'd like to use any of these to go beyond what's offered here, please feel free to do so, after you've become accustomed to the method.

The Method

A number of studies have established that the human brain, mind, and neurological system can't tell the difference between an event imagined in great detail and an event the body has actually moved through and perceived.[230] This is the basis for the effectiveness of visualization and imagery as a therapeutic method.

When applied to the healing processes of the body, imagery helps us to know that those healing processes are occurring, and so encourages them. When applied to the emotional issues that may be interrupting healthy function in the body, imagery helps us to restore the kind of function that makes it easier for the body to be healthy.

The method offered here is designed to encourage an experience of general well-being.

Introduction

As with all the methods described in this book, it helps to begin with Progressive Relaxation. We want the body to be as comfortable and uninvolved as possible as we allow the mind to do its work.

So find a comfortable place and position, preferably one in which you would not normally go to sleep. Make sure you're warm enough to sit for 15 - 30 minutes. You may want to have pencil and paper at hand to write down some of your experiences after you're done.

The Practice

Relax into your body. Feel it relaxing as you breathe.

Breathe in the nourishing air.

Breathe out any tensions or distracting thoughts.

Feel the body as it relaxes.

Feel the chest as it breathes.

Close the eyes if they're still open and rest them.

Feel the tension around them release.

Feel the air moving through the nostrils and throat.

Be aware that all is well as you begin this journey of self-care.

This is a comfortable and comforting thing to do.

This is natural and normal for human beings...

Simply relaxing and breathing,

Paying attention to the body in this moment, now.

Aware that the body is fully relaxed,

Now pay attention to the area in front of your closed eyes.

Notice that there is color and movement in your vision as you breathe.

Watch that movement for a moment, the colors or shapes,

Simply allow it.

And now, remember some beautiful place that you feel really comfortable in.

It may be a room or a park or a church or temple...

It may be some place you went hiking or fishing or camping...

Just remember a place where you feel good...

some place you enjoy.

Remember how it feels to be there

Remember the objects in that comfortable space,

The beauty,

The entrances, the exits,

The openings to the sky and places beyond.

The way the air felt against your skin, the scent of it in your nostrils...

Simply remember...

Remember going into that place and feeling good.

Remember relaxing there and being glad that you're alive and well when you're there.

Now feel yourself entering that space.

Feel the textures, see the colors, hear the sounds...

Simply enjoy being there for a little while..

Now be aware that someone is standing at the entrance to the space... someone that you trust, even if you don't remember seeing them before.

They're there to take you to another, even more wonderful place, even more wonderful than this...

And you realize you'd like to be in such a place

So you let yourself follow that person.

You're aware of moving through pleasant spaces, aware of pleasant sounds and colors, as you let that person lead you to another, even more wonderful place.............

And then, you become aware... you've arrived!

It feels wonderful!

The light and color are delightful as you look around and take it in with all your senses.

There's a soft music in the air, and you feel a gentle, warm breeze against your skin.

There's a place for you to sit and relax, to lie down if you choose, and you do so.

You feel yourself relaxing still futher

 into this wonderful-feeling space that you've been guided to.

Such peace...

Such joy...

It's as if you've truly come home.

And you breathe deeply in this relaxing, joyous space.

And the body relaxes further as you do so...

Please allow it to relax...

And you become aware that a wonderful, healing, beam of light is passing across your body...

You feel it as a loving touch as it glows on every part of your body with a healing ray

that restores full function,

balance,

harmony,

and well-being

to every cell and organ and tissue in your body.

You simply relax and breathe as you allow that loving light to restore your body, in this beautiful, joy-filled space.

Such beauty,

Such peace,

Such good feelings throughout the body

As you simply relax and breathe and take it all in.

And then the light fades and you realize the air is getting cooler and the sky is fading to dusk.

It's time to leave this beautiful place...

You allow yourself to look around

and you're aware that your guide is standing nearby and smiling.

You will be led safely back to your favorite space...

So you allow yourself to be guided back, feeling more alive, more alert than when you began this journey...

And when you return to the place you began, that wonderful, comfortable space that you remembered from before…

You look around, knowing you can come back here any time…

And with that thought your attention shifts…

You become aware of your breathing again…

you feel this body in this position in your normal space and time…

and you're aware that you're ready to move and stretch and breathe a few cleansing breaths…

Do so now, please…

Wiggle hands and feet and stretch and become centered once more in this body in this space and time, as you hear my voice…

Feel the renewed energy,

Feel the enthusiasm and delight as you open your eyes,

Fully awake,

Fully present,

Feeling better than ever!

Yes!

Now say it aloud, please: YES!

…as you sit up to write down whatever awareness you've received, or simply move on to the next part of your day.

ℰ

Releasing the Past; Healing the Present

Part of growing up and becoming an adult is learning to accept the events of our childhood and move on. Part of becoming healed is learning to release the decisions we made and the beliefs and memories we've hung onto, and freeing ourselves to move on. Part of freeing ourselves is learning how to discover those decisions and forgiving ourselves for having made them.

The process of discovering and letting go of the beliefs and ideas from the past, the "emotional hooks" that are driving our present experience is simple and powerful. Many therapeutic methods include aspects of it, but the full process is rarely taught.

The Method

This method is a synthesis of various techniques that, when applied to real, nondiagnosable health conditions, were found to be incomplete. Looking across many texts and practitioners, elements were found in some that weren't in others. What's been put together has been used with great success for years. It includes elements of traditional psychotherapy, spiritual healing, and a little of the 12-step program, as well as concepts from *A Course in Miracles*, and traditional guided imagery. This is the first time it's been published in this form.

The concept is based on the realization that Gabor Maté expresses so clearly in his *When the Body Says No*:

> The onset of symptoms or the diagnosis of a disease should prompt a two-pronged inquiry: what is the illness saying about the past and present, and what will help in the future?... What is not in balance? What have I ignored? What is my body saying no to?[231]

Another way of putting it is Florence Scovel Shinn's "It's not 'What's wrong with me?' but 'Who's wrong with me?'"[232]

Once we realize that our current experience is driven by the thoughts, beliefs, and fundamental assumptions that we hold in the cells of our body, then we have the potential for releasing them and moving on into full health and well being.

The process as outlined here, if done whole-heartedly and with as much feeling as possible, can release a very large portion of the stored energy and distress surrounding an idea that's been held in the body for decades. In the process, one may feel drained, elated, or overcome with feelings of longing, love, and grief. These are simply signs that long-buried feelings are coming to the surface to be freed. They're all good. And they're not permanent. They will pass. And that's good, too.

Doing this process can lead to a profound sense of freedom. People and situations that were once painful or otherwise distressing no longer even seem to occur, or if they do, it's far less intense. This state may last several weeks or months, until the old beliefs are "triggered" again, at a new level. At that point, even though it may feel as distressing as it has in the past, it's actually a much smaller level of distress that will last much less time (we like to say that each cycle through releases 80% of the stored energy). As soon as you become aware that you're in the old pattern again, simply do this process to release the next big portion (another 80% will take you down to 4% of the original power and duration—that's worth doing!) And so on, until you realize that the issue—and the behavior or symptom—is no longer in your life.

Introduction

This is an opportunity to put down a burden you've been carrying for a very long time.

This is a step into freedom.

This is the point at which the ideas and beliefs, thoughts and memories, that have driven your life for years can be let go of forever.

So find a place where you can have a few hours undisturbed and no one else will be disturbed by any sounds you may make or actions you may take.

Bring something to write with and some paper to write on—either scrap paper and pen or a chart pad and marker. You may wish to use a small recorder for some things, as well.

Releasing the Past; Healing the Present

Bring pillows and something safe to hit them with, if you should feel so inclined.

Bring a blanket or something to cuddle and be warm with.

Have a variety of music at hand—high energy dance music and soft, loving music—to listen to and support your process if you feel the desire.

Have plenty of water to drink and perhaps a light snack on hand, as well.

Now you can become the Self you were meant to be.

Before you start, simply state the intention that whatever you do or say is simply a form of release and will not be harmful for anyone or anything, anywhere.

The Practice

Sit comfortably and breathe. Pay attention to the situation that brought you to this place and time, doing this process.

Allow yourself to be aware of whatever is not working in your life or body right now.

Allow yourself to accept that this not-working, this not-okayness, this distressing experience, is what you've been experiencing.

Simply allow it.

Allow it and pay attention to it.

Please do this now...

Observe your experience:

What does it feel like? What are your thoughts saying?

What are you wishing?

Fearing?

Hoping?

Who comes to mind as you allow this experience?

Write down a few thoughts if you like, or speak them into your recorder, just so you know where you're starting, today.

Now, having become aware of what you're experiencing, accept that this experience is something you alone are experiencing.

Everyone else is having their own experience, and probably don't even know what you're going through, right now...

Accept then, that what you're feeling right now is not something you can blame on anyone else in the world around you...

they are not here...

they are not the reason you're feeling what you're feeling...

they're not thinking the thoughts you're thinking.

Accept that these thoughts are yours and yours alone.

Listen to them as they run through your mind: thoughts about yourself,

>   about others,

>   about the world.

Accept that these are your thoughts and they come from your mind,

And as you do so, realize that your mind generates them because of what it believes...

It's your own belief system that has generated these thoughts and these feelings.

Allow the feelings that come up when you hold that thought...

Feel the feelings and observe the thoughts...

You are the observer observing and the one who feels.

Again, accept that this experience and these feelings are not something caused "out there" but is a result of thoughts and feelings you've held "in here."

And with that, realize that while you may not be able to change what goes on "out there" you can definitely change what goes on "in here."

You are the one in charge of your thoughts, and so you can reduce or eliminate these feelings.

What power!

What possibilities!

You can be free of these feelings, these ideas, these beliefs that cause you such distress!

It's wonderful to know this, to accept this truth.

And it's important to realize that these ideas and beliefs—and the people who've showed them to you—have played an important role in your life. They have helped you become who you are, today—and that's really not all that bad!

Take a moment to honor the things you have accomplished in your life; the gifts others have received because of you; the things that are in place because of what you've done. Acknowledge that your life thus far has made a difference...

Because it has.

Now acknowledge that these ideas, this belief, these experiences and memories are part of why those things have happened... they have served you and you appreciate them...

But now it's time for them to go...

Just like graduating from high school or leaving home as an adult, it's not that you don't appreciate what was...

It's just time to put that way of thinking and being behind you and move on to something that serves you better, now.

So write or say aloud the sentence

"I acknowledge that these ideas have served me; they've brought me to this point in life; they've sometimes made it possible for me to do and be in ways I might not otherwise have been able. I am appreciative, but now it's time to let go of them and move on."

Notice what you feel as you say this…

What thoughts are going thru your mind now?

What kinds of anger or grief or frustration or fears are there?

What wants to be said that hasn't been said yet?

Allow these thoughts and feelings; write them down or speak them…

Shout them if you feel like it…

Sing them if that works for you…

Allow the feelings…

Some of them are running very deep, coming from very old places and memories…

Allow them to come…

Allow tears if they come…

Allow the arms and legs to move as they choose…

Allow whatever kind of language wants to be spoken… no one will be damaged by the words or the feelings. You are safe.

Allow them some more… there's a little more distress, sadness, pain hiding in there…

Let it flow…

let it move out of the mind-body…

It no longer serves you to carry this pain, these feelings in the mind-body, so let it go...

Write it if you like...

Hit something if you need to...

Imagine the people who taught you this or who kept this idea alive thru their actions and tell them everything you have ever wanted to say to them...

Write to them if it helps...

Now take a few moments to check in... is there more? what are the feelings now? What do you really want to say now?

Say it, whatever it is, knowing that no harm can come from letting it go...

Now check again: what thoughts and feelings are there?

When all you can think of to say is something like "I know you didn't mean to hurt..." or "I know you were doing the best you could..." or some such...

When your body feels drained and almost empty of energy...

Then you've completed expressing. You've "pushed from" the mind-body all that is available to let go now.

So breathe. Relax the body and breathe.

Feel the emptiness.

Feel whatever is there to feel...

Allow yourself to write or speak that it's done. You can use words like: "It's done. It's over. These ideas and feelings are released. They are no longer part of me or my world. I'm ready to release them and let them go."

Now allow the energy of the breath and that statement to help you

gather up anything you've been writing as part of this expression

tear it into little pieces, saying 'I'm done with this! It's no longer part of me!"

If you have a safe way to do so, now, burn that paper and watch it go up in smoke—if not, bury it or dissolve it in water—and as you do so repeat, "I'm done with these ideas! They are no longer part of my mind or body!"

Now allow yourself to imagine that you're holding a big vacuum cleaner and its sucking up all the energy in the space you've been using—all the words and feelings and pain and everything else that you've expressed—and clearing the air into a great big bag.

In your imagination, feel yourself tying off that bag and rolling it away from the space you're in. Imagine that it's disappearing... that it's imploding, or that some great loving being has come to transform it... You can even imagine that there's a rocket ship near by waiting to take off and you're rolling that bag up a ramp into the ship... to be fired off into the sun and transformed!

Feel the freedom of no longer having these thoughts, these ideas, running your life...

Now take a shower and allow the water to flow over your body, cleansing you...

Feel the energy of the water flowing through your body, removing the last little scraps of this stuff you've released...

As you get out of the shower, dry, and dress, know that you are done… It's over!

All that remains in you, and around you, is love and freedom and joy!

And in that awareness, sit down comfortably somewhere…

Sit and feel the feeling of love and freedom…

Breathe in that love, that freedom. Allow it to fill your mind-body.

As you do so, imagine that one of the people who were part of the pattern you've released is sitting in front of you…

The sense may be very clear or just sort of there—it doesn't matter.

Simply allow it…

Now say to that person all that you are thinking and feeling right now, about them, about the ideas you've released, about the possibilities for the future…

You may have only the fuzziest sense that they are there, or it may be very clear—it doesn't matter; just say what you have to say as if they were.

Now breathe…

And listen…

Listen inside you for whatever they may have to say to you… keep breathing…

keep listening… until you know you're done—they may or may not have something you need to hear, but you need to be open to it.

Please write down anything you learn in the process, then return to your breathing and relaxing and imagining this person is there with you.

Now tell this person that you've released the whole thing…

you're not holding on to it any longer…

it's not worth hanging on to…

effectively, you've forgiven them by letting it all go.

Observe your feelings… how does it feel to say that to them? Is there a little more to release or is it all clear?

If there's some hesitancy, some distress still there, simply imagine a new bag is beside you and that you can simply breathe out of your mind-body and into that bag any last little bit that's left. Lean over and do it now, please…

Now sit back and relax, breathing normally again, and with the person you've been imagining still there…

Speak to that person, saying something like, "I know we have some history around all this, but as I said, I've released it. So now I need to know that you're willing to let it go, too. Will you forgive me for hanging on to this so long?"

Again, listen with your inner hearing. Feel your feelings… allow whatever happens to happen.

If you have trouble understanding why you're doing this, remember: regardless of "who started it" you're the one who's been thinking all these negative thoughts all this time—that's what you're asking to have let go; that's what needs to be forgiven.

In all likelihood the person you're imagining will come back with some form of "yes." And as they do so...

Allow yourself to experience the beam of light that is now embracing both of you...

allow yourself to FEEL the forgiveness that is now and always was there available for both of you....

Feel the fact that you are totally forgiven... the universe, or God if you prefer, holds nothing against you... you are free!

Feel the freedom...

Feel the light...

Feel the love... embracing both of you...

Breathe it in and relax.

Now, feeling the love between you, declare how your future will be... what intention will you hold for both of you? What will you replace the old idea with?

Allow the images, symbols, and words to come. Write them or draw them if you like, and work with them until you have a clear statement. Then write that in the form of a present statement. Use whatever words come to you. If no words do, try something like "this person and I are complete and free from the past; we both go forth on our own paths in love and joy as we move forward in our lives."

After you've allowed the experience for one of the people you've been expressing about, give yourself a break. Go for a walk; have a light meal; do a fun dance—whatever feels like a pleasant way to occupy an hour or so. Or, if it's late, you may feel the need to sleep.

That's fine. Take care of you in whatever way feels good. ……….

When you're ready, come back to that comfortable spot and relax again…

Breathe…

And imagine the next person you've had issues with,

Repeat the above process with this person………………

Repeat it with the next…………………….

Repeat it with some of them in a group, if you like…

Allow yourself to experience total love and forgiveness with each and every one of them. You're letting go of a pattern that has imprisoned you and them!

Allow yourself to experience the freedom and joy of the State of Grace and Forgiveness, of Pure Beingness, without attachment to anything from the past.

Read the statements you've made regarding these ideas and these people…

Observe your thoughts and feelings now.

Make a commitment to read these every time you find yourself thinking any of those old thoughts and say "cancel" to those thoughts immediately if they come up.

You are free…

You are loved and loving…

You are surrounded by the light of compassionate awareness and totally safe and well…

Relax into and accept this truth of your being. For so it is.

Breathe 3 deep cleansing breaths and feel the energy moving through your body…

When you're ready, please pack up the things you've used in this space and give the space thanks for being there for you as you moved through this process.

You're ready to return to your "normal" life with a commitment to release anything that reminds you of that old set of ideas as they come up…

replacing them with the new declarations that you wrote as you completed with each of the people involved.

[In a few weeks you can repeat this process, when something like the old pattern comes up again, to get the next (much smaller) layer released.]

Compassionate Breathing
(Ton Len)

The various Buddhist traditions have given mind-body medicine some of its most useful methods, including powerful transpersonal methods. To the thousands of Americans studying meditation with Buddhist teachers, the practice of Ton Len, or Compassionate Breathing, was an essential practice by the time Sogyal Rinpoche published his landmark book, *The Tibetan Book of Living and Dying*. In the chapter called "Compassion: The Wish-Fulfilling Jewel," the method of Ton Len is published with full disclosure.[233] In Tibetan, Ton Len means "Giving and Receiving" or "Exchanging Oneself for Another." The practice has various applications as a transpersonal and self-care healing method.

In Tibet the practice of Ton Len was called the Holy Secret. The secret is exchanging oneself for another. It was used for both local healing and healing at a distance.

Dr. Larry Dossey has documented the numerous scientific studies of the effect of long-distance healing on others, whether or not they know that they are being "prayed for," or that healing energy is being intended to them. Yet beyond numerous anecdotal stories, we are not aware of any clinical trials focused on the dual healing benefits of Ton Len, Compassionate Breathing—studies needed to measure the doubly healing benefits of the practice, a practice that has remarkable self-care potential. It has been in use in cancer care, HIV-AIDS care, and hospice care since the 1970s, and in childbirth since 1997.

In cancer care, Ton Len has been used increasingly in the past twenty years because of its effectiveness. People can do the practice to abate their suffering and the suffering of others. A powerful use is when someone who has been lost in their suffering, say someone with AIDS or cancer, does this practice to give healing energy to another person with a similar condition. In so doing they forget their own suffering and practice being a healer.

When this method is given to cancer patients or AIDS patients, enabling them to practice the healing of another patient, it's wonderful to see someone who had been dwelling in suffering shift their attention and function to practice the healing of others.

This is what typically can happen (the following is a true story):

You are going to visit a woman dying of cancer in an oncology center. She is the mother of a friend of yours. You haven't met the woman. She knows that you're coming to visit her. She's alone in her room. She's glad that you've come. You ask her if she'd like a little massage on her neck and shoulders. She says she'd love that. She loves being caringly touched. You ask her how she is. She starts to describe her suffering. You breathe with her, in increasing communion.

Then you ask her if she'd like to do some meditation. She says, yes. She's never done that but she'd like to. You say that we're going to meditate with breathing. You ask her if she knows someone suffering from cancer as badly as she is. She pauses for a moment and then says, yes, she does know someone. You ask her to say that person's name aloud.

She does. You repeat the name. You say, Here's what we're going to do. Just forget your sickness. Part of you has always been well, has always been free. Right now, forget about being sick; just think about the person you've just mentioned. It doesn't matter how far away she is. You're going to reach that person instantly in your heart. This is more real and practical than probably anything you can imagine. You can practice the healing of that person with your breath.

Just breathe naturally, focusing into the sickness and suffering of that person. On your in-breath effortlessly breathe in all you can of that person's energy of sickness and suffering. Let it energetically come into the light in your body. That person's energy simply dissolves into your light. And effortlessly breathe out into that person all the energy they need to heal. You repeat the instruction once. You ask if she understands. She says 'yes.' Then you do the practice together. You feel the presence of the other woman. You and your friend's mother silently practice healing that woman. After a few minutes you realize that you're in the presence of something marvelous. The dying woman you're visiting has changed. She's become the practice of healing.

You continue the practice for about five minutes. It feels very powerful. You know that it's a remarkable event. The experience of a dying person compasssionately practicing the healing of another is unforgettable.

This is transpersonal medicine, universal field medicine. Because there is no separation of anyone or anything in the unified, universal field, you directly reach anyone in yourself, especially yourself. The practice can be done anywhere, anytime. We need only two things: the willingness to practice the healing of others by experiencing unlimited inherent healing energy in our systems, and the willingness to experience compassion, our natural ability to love, to do good.

No doubt it's healing for the spirit and mind of the sick person doing the practice, and it probably benefits the person the Compassionate Breathing is directed to.

Mother Teresa said it beautifully:

> Loving as He loves,
>
> Helping as He helps,
>
> Giving as He gives,
>
> Serving as He serves,
>
> Rescuing as He rescues,
>
> Being with Him twenty-four hours,
>
> Touching Him in his distressing disguise.[234]

Mother Teresa, like the Buddhist saints, embodied compassionate care. They gave us a great compassionate practice, at a time of great potential suffering and transformation.

The Method

MediGrace has developed a method of compassionate breathing called Transformative Compassionate Breathing. It's designed to assist anyone with the release and healing of any form of suffering—for oneself and for others.

In an age when there are probably more psychological disturbances than ever, and more undiagnosed and wrongly diagnosed disease conditions than ever before, we have, from perennial wisdom, a distinguished, proven method to spontaneously free us from conditioned states and, at the same time, enable us to effectively practice the healing of others.

Through compassion we give and we heal. Like thousands and thousands of people before you, you can do this practice. It's within your natural capability. Healing is basic to your life, basic to your life force. You are the healer who makes more than 50,000 different biochemicals, to dissolve potentially toxic substances that enter your body and to take care of all your internal needs. You are the life force that empowers your immune system. If you look into it, you may have unlimited healing energy. This is a gift that is yours to offer. You are being asked to use this gift, for your sake and for the sake of others. The practice can be applied to any disease condition.

In one of Shakespeare's most memorable passages he says:

> The quality of mercy is not strained,
>
> It drops as the gentle rain from heaven
>
> Upon the place beneath; it is twice bless'd;
>
> It blesseth him that gives, and him that takes . . .
>
> (Merchant of Venice, act IV, scene 1)

Even on one's deathbed one can turn away from being caught up in one's suffering. With this practice dying people turn freely to bless and heal others. With such a method it's relatively easy for a dying person to become a healer and a giver of blessings. Dying people can readily turn away from the conditioning of their life and enter the dynamic potential of the unconditioned state. Then the practice of Compassionate Breathing is genius, helping dying people heal into death.

Compassionate Breathing is therefore a perfect hospice method, for people working with the inner awareness of the comatose and others near death. Breathing effortlessly, we inhale the energy of sickness and suffering of that person's life, taking it in as if it were our own. It dissolves into light within, and we breathe out love and wisdom into the dying person. We bless that person and we are blessed by that person as we take in their suffering as blessing.

Introduction

First you do the practice for yourself, seeing your whole life at once, practicing compassion for yourself. It's immediately transformative since you do the practice from the light nature of your body.

If you are suffering a condition that needs healing, you first practice Compassionate Breathing for yourself.

Then, to heal yourself further, let go of the concept that you are suffering something that needs healing.

Drop that as completely as possible in order to practice healing someone else.

Forgetting yourself, with relief, you turn your focus to another person suffering the same sickness you have, or anyone suffering as much as you. You forget yourself and open your heart to the suffering person. You let go of who you think you are and what you think your body is.

Spontaneously you just follow your breath. Whatever your body is, it's just breathing naturally in and out. Opening yourself completely to the person who is suffering, on the in-breath you take in, you energetically breathe in, energy of the sickness and suffering of the other person, wherever they are. Effortlessly, with empathy, you take the energy of their suffering into yourself with your inhale, and you see that energy naturally dissolve into light in your body.

Effortlessly you breathe out into that person all the energy they need to heal.

What you inhale dissolves in light in you. You envision that the energy you send out, radiate out, intend out, heals and frees the other person of sickness and suffering.

In your intention to heal another person you activate healing in yourself. That is the essence of the magic. That is the practicality of the method.

If you do it sincerely you can and will experience how you can help others and heal yourself in the process.

In Compassionate Breathing, what we intentionally take in, we do not take on.

This is not psychic surgery.

We take energies of sickness and suffering into our light nature, into the multidimensional live light of our body.

We do not intentionally dissolve the energy of sickness into our light—

this is an important point.

We see that what we take in naturally dissolves into light in our body; we simply let it happen. We see that it is in our multidimensional nature that we cannot get sick, or be psychologically disturbed, by compassionately taking in the energy of sickness and suffering.

We are born to experience the energy of others' illness naturally dissolving into light in us.

And we effortlessly breathe out into others, or into our own body, the energy needed to heal and to evolve.

One can practice for oneself and another at once.

One can practice for several people at once.

The power of this practice cannot be overestimated, but of course that depends on the quality of our practice.

We can and should be fearless; that's a basis of any healing practice.

We do not manipulate what we take in.

We take it in energetically with unobstructed openness.

With this practice we can see, as tens of thousands of people have seen before us, that we are not "stuck with" our suffering, that it is our nature to let it go and to practice healing instead.

The instructions are traditional. They have proved effective through the ages. They are in increasing use in the medical establishment now.

The opportunity to express love, to express compassion, is healing for both oneself and for the one we express the compassion to.

In that double reality is true magic.

Traditionally you start by doing the practice for yourself.

Spontaneously sensing your whole life at once, shift into another dimension.

Enter your timeless universal nature

and see your life from your birth all the way through old age and death.

Seeing this as only you can, and as only you will know it,

feel deep compassion for yourself and your life.

Both because of all the suffering in the world

and because of many difficulties you probably have had,

open your heart to your self.

On your in-breath, without contriving your breath,

naturally breathe in whatever sickness and suffering you've had in your life.

Take it to heart.

See that it naturally dissolves into live light in you.

Then effortlessly breathe out into yourself all the healing energy you can use,

for any and every pain of mind, body, or spirit.

See that what you take in energetically dissolves into living light in you.

Now sense whatever future suffering you may have, and breathe it in.

See it all dissolve into your body light.

Effortlessly breathe out into yourself all the energy needed

to seal old and new wounds and calm your future pains.

Many, many people have healed themselves with this practice. The more you do the practice, the better the quality of your effort and the more alive the intention, and the more effective the practice will be.

Then do the practice for another, and then for more than one person at a time.

Please practice this method of healing, for yourself and for the world...

The Practice

You can do something for anyone who is suffering physical and/or mental distress,

yourself or anyone else.

You can practice Transformative Compassionate Breathing.

It's best to start with yourself.

Shifting into your timeless awareness,
sense your whole life deeply.

See your life from your birth through the present moment,
and sense the rest of your life.

Sense your whole life with compassion.

Following the natural flow of your breath, on your in-breath
effortlessly take in the energies of sicknesses and suffering
that you have had and will have. Simply take that all in,
in an empathetic response to your life.

The energy of distress and illness you take in
naturally dissolves into the light in your body,
and you effortlessly breathe out healing intention into your life.

Easily and completely, in the flow of your breath, all at once,
breathe in any remnants of traumas of your life, and at the same time
feel compassion for yourself for future and final challenges you'll face.

You inhale it and energetically take it into living light in you,
and as you breathe out, give out all the grace and compassionate energy you can use.

Please do this now. Breathe in and out with compassion this way.

You were made to be the healer of your life...

Turning to another person, someone you know well who has mental or physical torment, or both, someone your heart easily turns to, someone close to you,

in the natural flow of your breath, you effortlessly breathe in, take in

the energy of the disease, the torment, the crisis. It dissolves in live light in you,

and you effortlessly breathe out, intend out into that person

energies generated to reverse and heal their suffering.

You see that happen.

You see the energy go where it should go

and do what it should do.

Please do that now………………………………..

You easily breathe in, open-heartedly taking in the energy of someone's suffering,

someone you know, wherever they are.

What you take in dissolves into light alive in you,

and you breathe out, intend out

energies that can reverse and heal their suffering.

Please do that now………………………………………………

The longer you intend healing into yourself or into another
the more inevitable that healing will come.
Please practice that now.

You can shift from one person to another,
and you can practice Transformative Compassionate Breathing
for more than one person at a time.

Please do that now…………………………………

Breathe in, absorbing the energy of their anguish or sickness.
See that you can take it in easily and it immediately dissolves into light in you;
and breathe out healing energy into those people,
sensing their different conditions and needs.

No matter how much healing they need
you have that much to give and more.

Please practice your healing ability now………………

Turn to a hospital you know.

Imagine all its departments and services.

Imagine all the people coming there,
hoping for help with so many different conditions.

Sense the good intentions and the limitations of the hospital.

Sense how much more healing the patients need.

Follow the natural flow of your breath,
whether it is a short breath or a long one. Breathe with ease.
Understand that we live in a unified field.
Understand that the hospital is inside you.

Understand that you can breathe in, easily take in,
energies of the sickness and suffering in the hospital
with no chance of harming yourself,
and every chance of doing good.

Begin to know your unlimited nature.
Discover unlimited healing capability in yourself.

Practice the healing of everyone in the hospital at once.

Keep doing it until you feel the practice come alive.

Please do that now…………………………………

This is universal field medicine, transpersonal medicine.

You go beyond yourself, beyond what you think you can do,
and you do it because at last it's time to experience that.

It is time to know your deep healing ability.

It's time to know how much healing you can do.

It's time to know how much healing the world needs.

It's time to see that we touch the world more than we know.

It's time to practice healing touching all life.

Please do that now……………………………………

And so the time for this process is ending…
Take another deep breath and release the connection.
Breathe again and focus your attention on your own wellbeing,
as you move into the next phase of your own life.

ಏ

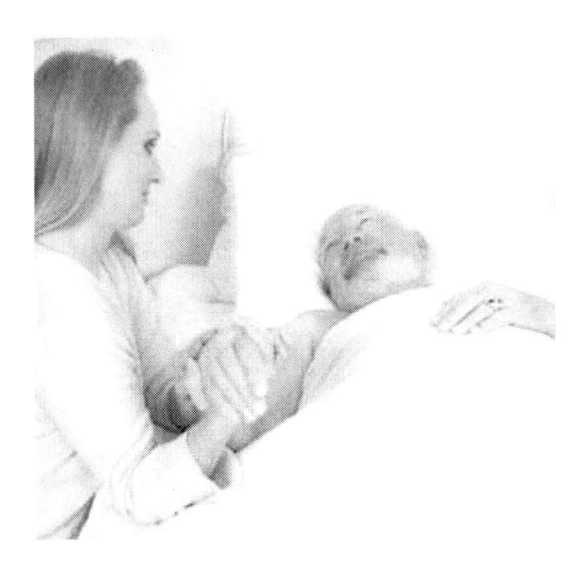

Caring for the comatose, semi-comatose, and those near-death—both caregiver and patient benefit from hearing the audioguide.

Healthcare Methods for the Semi-Comatose and Comatose, and for Near-Death Care

The methods presented so far are self-administered, typically using carefully recorded guided meditation. Such instruction makes it possible for anyone to achieve the healthful effects of deep meditation anywhere, without years of training or discipline. And, importantly, recorded audio-guides provide a means for practicing self-care methods regardless of the capacity of the listener to speak or act. Administered to the comatose or dying, the audio-guides help the patient maximize inner awareness to restore balance, when outer concerns and capacities no longer seem to matter.

Guidance to inner awareness may enable people to shift states. It may cause release into unconditioned being. It may not be possible to see the effects of the audio-guides with ordinary observation, but when quality efforts are made to reach the inner awareness of patients in nonresponsive states, that care has done something important for them. A few of those people may have remarkable results, whether we know it or not.

The healing that may occur with these methods is not always visible to the eye but is usually felt. As we observe those who are no longer able to communicate with us verbally respond to these practices, we can sometimes see them relax into a new state of being, but even if we don't see changes, we may feel them. Those we love and care for are not from us; they are in the energy body we are. As we still our minds and sense the one whose manifest body is so still, we may sense the shift that the life goes through when the heart stops and the inner light brightens.

The following methods apply audio-guide meditation in a variety of settings. The assumption is that someone is reading these treatment texts aloud, or that there's a speaker placed near the person being treated with a recording playing for several hours a day.

1. ALZHEIMER'S CARE: TREATMENT FOR THE SEMI-COMATOSE

Over the past decades, Alzheimer's disease has become a significant, expensive healthcare problem, destroying the lives of millions of elderly individuals and placing immense stress on their families, particularly the primary caregiver. The disease progresses slowly, sometimes affecting the lives of those involved for as much as a decade. Its characteristic symptoms are:

- memory loss
- general cognitive dysfunction
- dementia
- autism
- increasing physical dysfunction

In spite of many millions of dollars spent in research, experimentation, and treatment, Era I medicine, with its focus on the chemistry and physiology of the body and brain, has failed to either prevent or treat this sadly debilitating condition.

However, the potential for healing through direct access to inner awareness is great. By focusing on the function that underlies all mental processes, it's possible to reduce, and even reverse, many symptoms. The torment many patients feel, knowing that they can't speak or think as they used to or want to, can be released as they turn away from trying to deal with the outer world and turn inward to inner awareness, to deep, inner knowing in the nonverbal, transpersonal domain.

This remarkable true story is an inspiration for our approach to Alzheimer's therapy. Published in *Kitchen Table Wisdom*, by Rachel Naomi Remen, the story is told by a doctor, Tim, about his father. About ten years before his death, Tim's father had become silent and then progressively more passive and helpless, requiring constant care. One day, Tim's mother had gone shopping and Tim and his brother, fifteen and seventeen years old, respectively, were watching a football game on TV, with their father seated in a chair nearby. Suddenly, there was a loud crash. Their father had fallen forward heavily onto the floor. His face was gray; they knew something was seriously wrong. Tim told his brother to call 911. Then a voice they hadn't heard for ten years said, "Don't call 911, son. I'm all right. Tell your mother that I love her." And he died.[235]

Similar anecdotes about the comatose and semi-comatose abound, pointing to an inner awareness and capacity that seem impossible when brain function has so badly deteriorated. There are many such remarkable stories, and for every one that is reported, research has shown that up to a hundred similar stories go unreported. Carl Jung said that of all the clinical experience he had in his career, his observation of a persistent subjective state in cases of severe damage to the cerebral cortex or in states of brain "collapse" was most remarkable. He saw it as evidence of a possible persistence of consciousness after death. [236]

Recent studies indicate more clearly than ever the need for methods to reach the inner-awareness of those in vegetative states. In one study, Adrian Owen and coworkers in the U.K. asked a patient in a vegetative state to think of certain mental images ("Imagine playing tennis" or "Imagine visiting the rooms in your house"). The resultant brain activation was no different from that observed in healthy control subjects, suggesting that some people in a vegetative state are more conscious than we realize. This technique was used to communicate with four out of 23 vegetative patients who would otherwise have been considered unconscious....Over the last few years, brain imaging studies like Owen's, along with other projects, have improved our tools for studying consciousness.[237]

The Method

The method we are presenting here was developed by MediGrace to therapeutically access inner awareness. An audio-guide is available on the MediGrace.org website, Alzheimer's Care (MG5). It provides direct access to inner awareness through the use of an audio-guide, giving instructions to shift attention to inner awareness..

This method has a twofold healing potential: it reduces stress and supports the inner foundation for mental and physical functioning, in both the patient and the caregiver, at the same time. For the most beneficial impact, we recommend that both the patient and caregiver have regular opportunities to listen to the audio-guide together.

Since the caregivers will be applying the method for themselves as well as for the patient, this is both self-care and administered care.

Introduction

Following is a condensed version of the audio-guide transmission of the method. A full version is available on the Medigrace cd #MG3, *Calm Healing*.

The Practice

And so we sit here, quietly,

breathing.

Let's breathe together.

Let's be quiet together.

Let's feel the energy

in the inner quiet.

Let's learn peace.

Let's breathe together.

Let's have this quiet.

Let's learn peace.

Teach me to communicate

with you in a new way.

Teach me to find your wisdom inside.

Teach me to find
the inner way.

Look at me
from your inner mind.

Communicate telepathically.

Let me hear you
without listening.

Let me know you
without thinking.

Let me see you
without looking.

I'm letting you reach me
from deep inside you.

Reach me
from the life you can't express.

Teach me
to be telepathic.

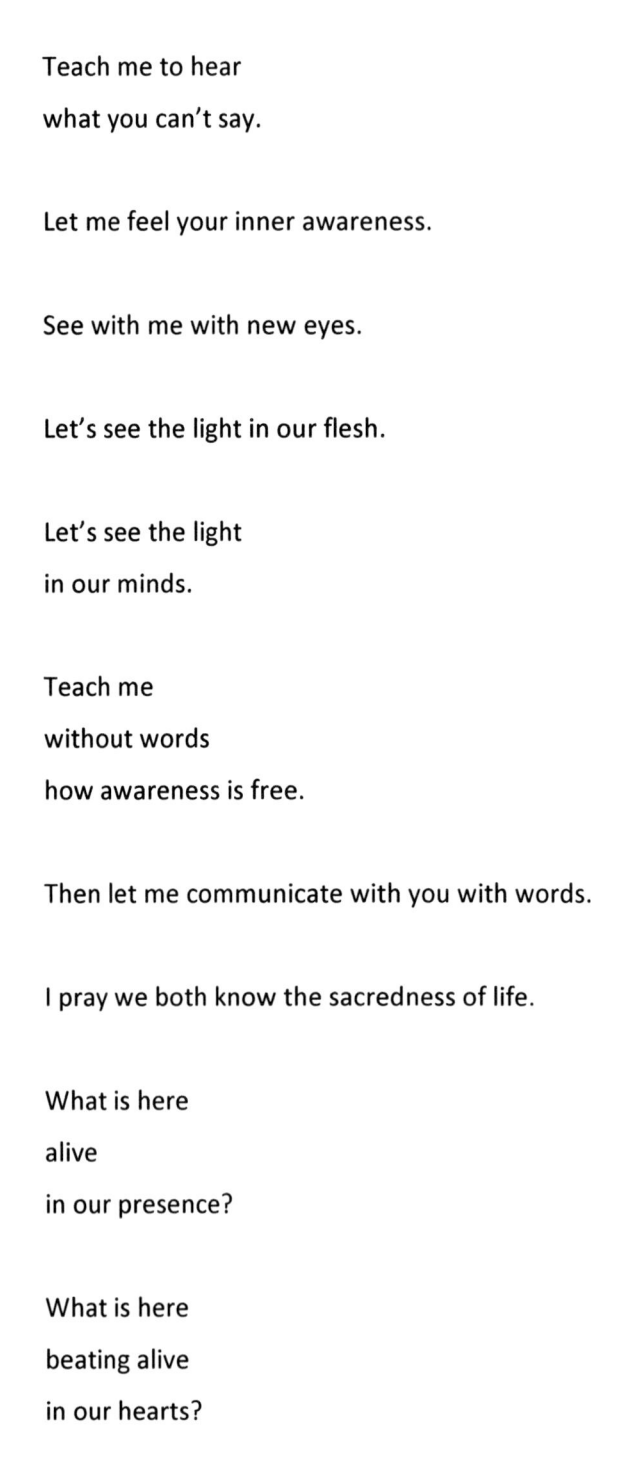

Teach me to hear
what you can't say.

Let me feel your inner awareness.

See with me with new eyes.

Let's see the light in our flesh.

Let's see the light
in our minds.

Teach me
without words
how awareness is free.

Then let me communicate with you with words.

I pray we both know the sacredness of life.

What is here
alive
in our presence?

What is here
beating alive
in our hearts?

Heal with me into grace.

Now is the time
to turn into
the source of life.

Understand me when I express my care,
and show me again how much you care.

Could it be
that we hold
the key to peace?

Without words
show me inside
your open mind.

Let's be quiet now
and touch the pulse of life.

Let's reach new ways to meditate inside.

Let's now go so far into life
we'll come into the presence
of the depths of life,
awareness itself.

Let's be alive
in this secret place
to realize peace,
joy and peace.

Sit with me now.

Breathe with me now.

Let's bless the world.

Let's be in peace.

2. CARE FOR THE COMATOSE

In altered states such as coma, the patient may be, or seem to be, "stuck" in an impenetrable isolation. But since the West has discovered inner awareness and the possibilities associated with nonlocal mind,[238] some of us have shifted our attention to the inner awareness of those in such states, beginning to explore ways to reach people who once were believed to be unreachable. In some cases, we are able to help them shift attention sufficiently to break out of states that have locked them away from the outer world. As Arnold Mindell observes,

> We are less concerned with recovering expression or movement than with facilitating inner release and realization . . . refine methods to help people in altered states connect to their own inner awareness.[239]

Though words in the audio-guide call those who will hear them to "come to life," to "regain life," it'st to be understood from the way it's being said that the text is not necessarily calling for the listener to awaken from the comatose state, or to reverse the process of dying. If that happens, good; if not, a level of healing and inner release has been encouraged. The "life" that the reader's voice is calling one into is beyond the material body. It's the inherent awakened state, what Arnold Mindell has called "the immortal you...

> ...Life after death appears as a timeless eternal reality trying to manifest itself in the pesent.[240]

Death can be a healing into greater life, as many have discovered.

The Method

Understanding this possibility, and on the basis of the research concerning awareness-based meditation techniques, MediGrace has developed an audio-guide, "Healing Through Hearing in Unconscious States" (MG2, Side A), combining language and music to help people in altered states develop their capacity to function in inner awareness. Designed to reach inner awareness and offer the possibility of release, or even realization, the audioguide may be used in routine nursing care or in-home care.

The following script is provided so that you may create your own audio-guide.

Introduction

The audio-guide is most effective when played at a soft, but audible sound level, near the patient's head. We can be confident in the knowledge that there are ways to guide people in profoundly altered states, such as coma, to a new sense of life and possibility.

The Practice

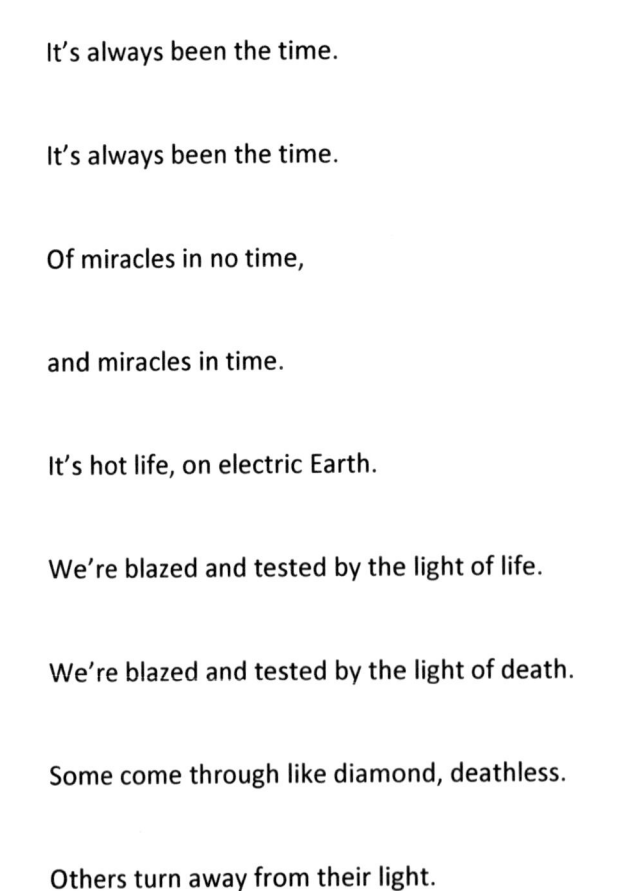

It's always been the time.

It's always been the time.

Of miracles in no time,

and miracles in time.

It's hot life, on electric Earth.

We're blazed and tested by the light of life.

We're blazed and tested by the light of death.

Some come through like diamond, deathless.

Others turn away from their light.

Some break through all interference

and their life dynamic takes charge.

Life force comes alive in them.

They come alive inside.

They are a force of change.

This is music for a new kind of sight.

This is music for a new kind of speech.

This is music for a new kind of life.

You can hear it in the action you beat.

You can go into the goodness of your light.

There's no stopping the world from evolving.
There's no stopping the life the new world has to give.

Earth is absolutely charged with life,

and it pulses with the charge into space.

This is music for a new charge of life.

This is music for a new vital blaze.

Come to life awake.

Blaze with life awake.

Blaze inside out.

Now is the time.

Now is the time.

It's always been the time of the miracles of life.

It's always been the time of the miracles of death.

We're always tested by the light of life.

We're always tested by the light of death.

Some have to break through now.

Break through into light.

It's still not too late.

Some break through all their blocks

and their flesh comes alive with light.

The force of it heals body and mind.

This is compassion of the clear light field.

Now is the time to see.
.
Now is the time for greater life.

This is music for new life in your mind.

This is music for new life in your face.

The action in your cells changes fields.

You come clear in the live charge of your heart.

You are more and more charged with life.
You pulse with the charge to awake.

This is music for a new charge of life.

This is music to awake the state.

Come to life
gaining charge.

Come to blaze

receiving life.

Awake at last,

wake for good,

once and for all.

3. HEALING IN NEAR-DEATH CARE

The hospice care movement emerged at the end of the twentieth century, during the height of Era I medicine—an era that has been characterized by the intensive use of drugs, machines, and other medical techniques to intervene in and extend the final stages of bodily life. With the emerging Era III understandings of the nonlocal effects of practices such as the Buddhist Ton Len (see Chapter Ten), hospices now can offer new possibilities for people completing the life cycle.

Meditation-based near-death care prepares people for the powerful experiences they will encounter as the body begins to shut down, and offers new ways to help people previously thought to be out of reach achieve new levels of capability.

The Method

Audio-guidance in near-death states can facilitate inner awakening and the realization of deathless states as the body seems to be letting go of life. The MediGrace audio-guide "Near Death Care/After Death Care" (MG2, Side B) may be self-administered or administered by a caregiver.

Potential applications for this method include:

- anyone wanting to do healing work while asleep (self-administered)
- anyone who is bedridden and largely unconscious or comatose due to late stages of a disease (administered)
- anyone whose brain has been traumatized (administered)
- anyone preparing for death and rebirth (administered and self-administered)

This audio-guide method may be used for inner development at any time in life, and in hospice care. It may be applied in routine hospital nursing, in-home care, or hospice. It is applied to the incapacitated person at soft but audible sound levels near the person's head. The combination of voice and sacred sound is intended to reach inner awareness, offering the possibility of inner release or even liberation, a healing of the spirit.

Though words in the audio-guide call those who will hear them to "come to life," to "regain life," it's to be understood from the way it's being said that the text is not necessarily calling for people to awaken from comatose states, or to reverse states of dying, and arise. If that happens, good; if not, a level of healing and inner release may still have occurred. The "life" that the recorded voice is calling one into is life beyond physical life and death, the inherent awakened state, what Mindell calls "the immortal you....

Life after death appears as a timeless eternal reality trying to manifest itself in the present".[241]

Death can be a healing into greater life, as many have known.

Introduction

In the immediate moments after death we can hear in two ways. We not only hear very clearly, because the mental body has all the faculties of the physical body, but we telepathically know the meaning of the sacred texts that may be read to us. And, according to anecdotal evidence, we are able to practice the teachings as we hear.

The MediGrace audio-guide "Liberation Through Hearing After Death" (cassette #MG2, Side B) is a concise presentation of the Bardo prayers of *The Tibetan Book of the Dead* (more literally translated, "The Great Liberation Through Hearing in the Bardo"). It is all based on that sacred text.

The words invoke awareness directly, instructing us to realize our light, now and in the after-death states. The instructions are offered before and after death, understanding that even after death we have chance after chance to come alive. Awakening to awareness at any time is transformative, even in altered states of being.

The audio-guide gives famous sacred instructions for dying and for progress in the after-death states. The program has been edited for general use in homes and in hospices. It is administered at a low, but audible volume, either with headphones or speakers placed very near the head. The program begins with an introduction to the Tibetan text.. This is a famous revelation of Padmasambhava, who brought Vajrayana Buddhism to Tibet in the ninth century. It's a major subject of Sogyal Rinpoche's *The Tibetan Book of Living and Dying*. Then the music begins, an ancient music for many instru-

Treatment for the Semi-comatose & Comatose, and Near-Death Care

ments, great horns and drums, resonant with harmonies of the greater world. It makes a timeless field for the melodic chanting of the revered instructions, teachings said to liberate when they are heard.

This is a melodic energy medicine applied when conventional, Era I medicine can only obscure, distress, or disturb natural processes that could lead to transformation or transcendence. This method gives us something special to offer to those who are dying and those who have just passed on.

Following is a version of the audio-guide transmission of the method. You can obtain the audio-guide and experience the method through audio-guidance or use this script.

The Practice

And so you will come to the death of your physical body,

your time to enter a new state of being.

Let's make an offering of music,

awakened music,

and let's hear the sacred instructions,

called Liberation Through Hearing After Death.

During the time of life in this human body

few people succeed in waking up.

In physical death and in states after that

we have chance after chance to come alive.

This is what ancient wisdom is saying.

Before and after death listen to the sacred instructions.

We have the chance to awaken again and again after death.

After physical death we're much more clairvoyant,
more in touch with light.

After death we have great understanding and knowing.

After we die we can
read the mind of a living person.

We can hear telepathically,
understanding the meaning of a text read to us,
even if we've never heard the language before.

The ancient wisdom says that in states after death
the mental body has the faculties of the sense body.

We're told that we can see and hear intently after death.

We can be invoked to hear and realize the wisdom teachings.

But just as intensely our mind projects and interferes.

The great challenge after death is to recognize mind,

to be much more aware.

So prepare to be awake as your body dies,

awake in death.

Recognize mind.

Be ready to receive all-knowing teachings.

Be ready to be sane and free.

So now, at whatever moment of your life

you can use teaching on how to recognize mind,

and how to act for the benefit of all life.

Especially when we're close to the time of death,

in order to prepare for the intensity of being disembodied,

or if we are now in an after-death state,

hear the music and the voice of the wisdom teachings.

Hear and become liberated for the benefit of all life.

PART FOUR: NEW POSSIBILITIES

One of the more profound consequences of using the methods outlined in Part Three of this book is that we begin to realize that our distress and pain are not burdens to bear, but opportunities to transform. As we use the breathing and the compassion and the healing processes contained in these methods, we begin to see that we are not the illness, nor the body in distress. We begin to understand that we are not the victim of some dreadful organism or circumstance or system. And, as we begin to experience freedom from all these limited perceptions, we begin to move through and beyond the symptoms that required us to stop and use the methods in the first place.

Transforming Our Paradigm of Illness & Wellness

Historically, Era I medicine has focused on applying a particular protocol to an individual with particular symptoms. The assumption was that, at best, that individual would be free of those symptoms and, at worst, that individual would continue to suffer or the symptoms would cause him or her to die, at which point the medical practitioner would simply try to make a patient pain free as he or she moved through the dying process. Yet more and more evidence tells us that this need no longer be the case.

The Genius & Potential of Self-Care

The genius of self-care is that the patient applies it from within, accessing inner resources that may have been previously unused. Even if the patient has intentionally used inner resources for healing to some degree in the past, he or she may not have begun to access them deeply. It's a rare person who has accessed their inner resources enough to know that they may be unlimited.

The genius of self-care is that most people can access inner resources to heal or mitigate most health conditions, and can change their lives for the better in the process. How much any individual may be able to heal a specific health problem depends on three factors: the availability of proven self-care methods; education in the use of the methods; and the quality of effort the person gives to the use of the method.

Self-care methods do exist in the public domain today. Through the unfolding of remarkable historical processes, a significant number of people on our planet, enough to make an important difference in human evolution, have access to methods that can restore healthy body function and transform consciousness. The question is: will forces of history compel the corporate medical stronghold to allow self-care into the center of the medical paradigm in the near future? We need that change soon, for the sake of human health, for the sake of the evolutionary quality of the species. The fact that educators and the general public are asking for changes in the field of medicine based on human needs and rights is evidence of a positive historical force.

Self-care is the heart of Caroline Myss' revolutionary proposal to transfer power from the doctor to the patient. Self-care is the central feature in Herbert Benson's vision of what the medical paradigm must become. Everyone has an inherent right to use self-care methods for general medicine, and for the transforming experiences of birth and death. Every woman has the right to be educated in advanced natural childbirth methods, self-care methods that may bring out her innate ability for higher levels of prenatal and postnatal care. Everyone has the right to experience the transformational potential in illness. And, in the final stages of life-in-the-body, everyone has the right to be educated in near-death care methods that facilitate the transformation of consciousness as body functions cease. Every man, woman, and child has the right to be educated and trained in Progressive Relaxation and full, imagery-enhanced, optimal breathing—the essentials for well-being in all anxiety-ridden situations.

It's time to call for greater education in the potential of self-care methods. Everyone has the right to be educated and trained in healing meditation methods—to experience the genius of self-care. It's time to propose new healthcare education in which people are encouraged to use self-care as a primary option. Education is the key.

Opportunities

Earlier, we suggested that illness is a state of consciousness. We outlined some of the characteristics of that state, including the fact that people tend to become passive, rather than active, moving in and out of sleeping/dreaming more frequently than in "normal" waking consciousness. Interestingly, it is in these subconscious shifts that the opportunity for transformation of consciousness is found.

As we find ourselves less active, we are more willing to relax. As we find ourselves more "dreamy" and less "focused," we are more willing to simply observe our breathing and the thoughts that move through our awareness. As we feel more discomfort in our body, we are more willing to find ways to release the sensation. As we drift into the inner dimensions of semi-coma, we process and release the past with fewer distractions from the present.

Western scientific medicine has seen these characteristics of illness as symptoms to be treated or, at best, stages in the healing process. Across time and cultures, only the shamanic traditions, based on the understanding that all of life is a balancing of interacting forms of consciousness, have treated illness as a state of consciousness to be transformed by the practitioner. In our culture, only "faith healers" and Christian Science or New Thought practitioners have done so. The fact that this approach works (for example, Science of Mind practitioners must have 3 documented healings to earn their license) has not prevented Western science from calling such practitioners "witch doctors" and "charlatans," simply because the observed results haven't fit the materialst scientific paradigm.

Today, however, with the new understandings of how matter and energy are formed and transformed, and with the undeniable results of thousands of experiments showing the nonlocal nature of mind, it is ignorance to discount the effectiveness of mental and energetic approaches to illness. So western researchers are in the middle of a scientific revolution—a shift from a paradigm of analysis and deductive reasoning based on materialst assumptions and toward a paradigm of holism and intuitive understanding.

Fortunately, a few experts in the "new" paradigm remain. A few "medicine men and women" and "holy men and women" and swamis and yogis and lamas and shamans have managed to continue their practice and teaching in ways that Westerners can learn and benefit from. We have relied on these teachings for this book. Our model of the human mind-body in Part Two and the methods suggested for use in Part Three are derived and integrated from both the new sciences and the ancient wisdom.

And, as we have done so, we've seen our own understanding transformed. For we, like so many others in our culture, had tended to see illness as something to avoid, something to heal and move on from. But as we worked with and practiced and thought about our experience with these ideas and the methods, we came to understand that, through the experience of illness, each of us (and the people around us) had gone through a transformative process.

Transformative Processes

One way to look at this process is presented in C. S. Holling's ecosystems model. Holling, a biologist trying to understand the dynamics of insect infestations in forests, has described a process that applies to all living systems in distress.

According to Holling, everything starts as a seed—an idea, a dream, an egg. The seed grows and develops and becomes a seedling, a vision, or a company or an activity. This grows and includes more and more others—cells, plants, animals, or people—and begins to take on structure. The structure gets stronger and stronger: the tree no longer sways with the wind, the company no longer reacts to the market, the body no longer bounces back as quickly.

Then some shift occurs in the environment. It may be major, a storm or fire or job loss, or it may be seemingly minor, like a change in the cost of a raw material or the minimum wage. But the structure is so inflexible that the change is too much. There's no easy way to respond, so it begins to fall apart. Things get chaotic. Trees fall down. Companies go under or cut way back. Bodies get high fevers or weird growths.

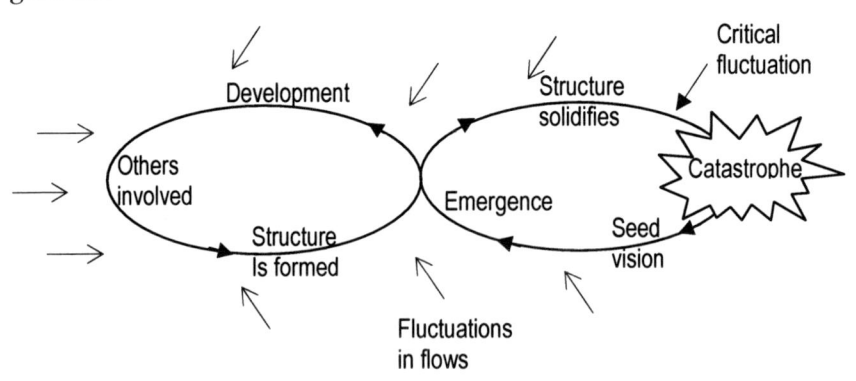

C. S. Holling's ecosystems transformation model, simplified.

Then, remarkably, in the midst of the chaos, something happens. New seeds emerge (the seeds of redwood trees and some grasses need fire to sprout!). New ideas can be implemented that couldn't have existed before. New relationships are formed. So the cycle begins again. Nothing is quite the same, but the same process happens anyway—until the next "catastrophe" and ensuing "chaos" allow new seeds to form.

Illness goes through the same process. In fact, virtually every state of consciousness can be seen as going through the same process. More interestingly, however, illness is usually seen as the "catastrophe" and the "chaos" in the process of our lives—disrupting normality with its demands and distress and too often leaving a path of destruction in its wake.

Yet if we know that this process is how life works and we think of illness as the result of a "catastrophe" that has led to this "chaos" out of which new seeds will emerge for our lives, then a whole new set of possibilities opens up for us. Now, instead of wasting our energy being upset at the symptoms, we can be grateful for the opportunity to rest. Now, instead of being upset at the disruption of our routine, we can appreciate the new perspective that being still for a while can give us. Now we can carefully and patiently observe the symptoms to see what the mind-body is telling us through them—what kinds of needs have not been met; what kinds of actions might be taken. Now, instead of making a big deal out of our own distress, we can use the opportunity to consider the distress of others and begin to be compassionate (from the root meaning "feeling with").

If we go beyond the immediate experience and consider how it has emerged through our history, we can see the opportunity for empathy and a deeper relation to oneself. If we go into the immediate present and, using methods like those presented in this book, allow ourselves to experience the depths that are possible in meditation, we can use the opportunity provided in illness to experience pure awareness or *rigpa*, that state beyond time and space which is complete sanity, primordial sanity. Such a state is found in quiet and rest. It's inborn.

So illness can be a transformative process, turning things around, a revolution. To be aware of what's happening, in order to help yourself, you need to find psychological freedom. When you're more aware of subconscious and paranormal currents in your systems, you may directly sense that the purpose of life is to realize your potential. Illness may enable us to see that self-care can be transformative. Illness may, indeed, as so many people have reported, start us on the path to true realization.

Healing the Person, Healing the Planet

In these pages we've developed a model of the human mind-body that is far more than the material structure most of us have been trained to focus on. We've used this model to explain how it is that the body can be healed by intentional mental and emotional activity—and particularly through various forms of meditation.

We've explored the body of healing methods called "transpersonal" and even provided a couple of methods that draw on transpersonal potential.

But we have not, as yet, explained how they work, or what their potential is for human experience.

The Transpersonal Mind-Body

How it is that what one person thinks or feels can affect another's sense of wellbeing has been a focus of interest for humanity throughout the history of Western culture. Because industrial culture (in whatever language or location), unlike most other cultures, believes that each human being is isolated and separated from everyone else by the skin, the mechanism for transpersonal processes has historically eluded our scientific thinkers. In cultures that see each human being as part of a universal "web of life" or "spirit," this is not a problem. For them, what is experienced anywhere within the web is communicated everywhere—one simply has to learn how to read the signs.

Lacking such a perspective, and required by the traditions of science to use only measurable data as indicators, Western researchers have attempted for generations to develop theories that explain what they have observed—and, often, experienced: the direct apprehension of another person's thought or feeling. Typically, as in the Western esoteric tradition, they have found it impossible to do so within the scientific-materialist paradigm. As Alan Watts stated in one of his last seminars, "We spend the first year of our life learning that the self ends with our skin and the rest of our life trying to unlearn it."

As we've seen, however, the field of transpersonal studies has offered a number of scientifically validated descriptions of the transpersonal experience. Transpersonal researchers have demonstrated beyond question that people and events can affect our thoughts, emotions, and even our illnesses without physical interaction—even at a distance. Michael Murphy has thoroughly documented in *The Future of the Body* hundreds of experiments and research results that support the realization that there are dimensions of the human experience that transcend the limitations of the physical, material body.

Rupert Sheldrake's work, described in *The Sense of Being Stared At*, is an attempt to apply the rules of controlled experiments to the anecdotal observations of thousands of people who have responded to his requests. He has demonstrated statistically that people are aware more ofteh than not when someone focuses attention and perception toward them, and that they can sometimes tell when someone is about to telephone or email them.

Itzhak Bentov, in his *Stalking the Wild Pendulum*, offers an explanation. Based on the model of the mind-body system as a set of overlapping wave forms, he suggests that as our "observers," or information waves, are periodically expanding into the inner torus of the universe, so are the "observers," or information waves, of everybody else:

> For a tiny fraction of a second we form an information hologram with them, and this is repeated many times a second... our psyches, which contain all our knowledge, expand periodically into that space for a very short period of time at practically infinite velocities. There the human psyches form an interference pattern with the psyches of all other consciousnesses in the universe. This interference pattern, or hologram of knowledge-information, we can call the "universal mind."... We can't separate global mind from universal mind...[242]

This has profound implications for understanding the nature of interpersonal interaction. The energy field of, for example, a teacher or healer with whom we resonate may affect our own fields with healing and integrative energy that interacts with ours to create a new

Healing the Person, Healing the Planet

level of functioning—which is the traditional explanation for darshan or satsang in the Hindu and Sikh traditions of teaching and learning. In another case, the energy field of a family member, coworker, or supervisor that is not in resonance with our own can negatively affect our mood and, sometimes, our level of function.

The recognition of our transpersonal nature also has implications for understanding our own experience of self. If "who I am" is affected by the thoughts and feelings of those around me—and those distant from me whose energy fields can reach me quickly by email or phone—then what is "who I am"? Can I consider myself a separate individual, especially when I feel my universal energies?

Transpersonal therapists say "No." They see what perennial wisdom has been seeing, that our personal life is limited, and constantly changing, but our transpersonal life is unlimited and healed in the great unified field. In this aspect, the transpersonal model is very like the Buddhist model, with its Dharmakaya and Sambhogakaya bodies as aspects of the human mind-body experience. It's also very much in alignment with the "fields within fields" model of human energetic systems that we described earlier. Clearly, an integration of these models is possible.

An Interconnected Whole

The tools and ideas offered by *The Whole Earth Catalog* through the late 1960s and into the '80s planted the seeds of a sustainable global culture in the popular mind, but Theodore Roszak's *Person/Planet*, published in 1979, was perhaps the first description of the practical implications of living in a media-based "global village." Fritjof Capra followed with his *The Web of Life*, which provided a systems-based framework for understanding the interconnected organism that is the biosphere. As we described in the chapter on Models of the Mind-Body system, Rupert Sheldrake has continued to develop his work with Morphic Resonance since the original publication of *A New Science of Life* in 1981, suggesting that some form of information field surrounds the planet, affecting the tendencies of events at the levels of the organism and cells.

Through these and many other syntheses of ideas and theories, we can observe a rich pattern of field-based understandings emerging, helping those of us who live in Western Industrial culture see that we cannot be isolated.

Quantum Relationship

Another approach to understanding the nature of our interconnectedness has emerged from the field of quantum physics. Though the work and ideas of Fred Alan Wolfe (*Space-Time and Beyond; Quantum Reality*), Nick Herbert (*Quantum Reality*), and Brian Greene (*The Elegant Universe*) are perhaps best known, a remarkable series of books by Oxford physicist-philosopher Danah Zohar provides a useful perspective. Zohar, whose husband is a psychotherapist, was writing books explaining quantum processes when she became pregnant. As she went through the process of nurturing the life within her, she became aware that she was no longer able to identify herself as an isolated individual. She had to acknowledge that her identity was no longer that of an isolated entity but was a function of her relationships. She proceeded to write *The Quantum Self*, which was soon followed by *Quantum Society* and later, with her psychiatrist husband, *SQ: Connecting with Our Spiritual Intelligence*.

Zohar's thesis is that the fundamental units that make up all matter and energy in the universe are neither matter nor energy but, in fact, tendencies for relating. These minute "wavicles," far smaller than electrons or even photons, emerge and then disappear into and out of nowhere.

One of these is the boson, named after Satyendra Nath Bose, the physicist from India who partnered with Einstein to describe the Bose-Einstein condensate. It's the basis for superconductivity, a quality by which a piece of matter is instantaneously and wholly affected by anything that happens to any part of it. Zohar says the boson is the tendency to come together. The recent scientific fervor over the determination that the Higgs Bozon actually exists is the final proof of the model that says every particle of matter arises from a tendency to come together within the universal quantum field.

The second, the fermion (named after the Italian American who led the Manhattan Project that first split the atom, Enrico Fermi), is the tendency to move apart. Every form of energy emerges out of this tendencay to spread apart.

All aspects of the universe are made up of these two manifestations of the quantum vacuum, as they interact in a dynamic balancing act in the formation of energy and matter.

Zohar suggests, that these, along with electrons and photons, make choices to act as matter and energy and so exhibit a rudimentary form of intelligence that is present everywhere, always, throughout the universe. This intelligence, she says, increases with the complexity of the system they compose. She calls this intelligence, or consciousness, "panpsychism." Then she offers a model of life that is made up of increasingly complex, interrelated fields of energy-based consciousness, centering on apparently individual organisms, which exist only in terms of their interrelatedness with other such patterns of energy/consciousness. She concludes with the revelation that we human beings must then exist only in terms of our relationships with other.

Itzhak Bentov, coming from another perspective, agrees: Matter contains/is consciousness. Our planet is therefore a larger consciousness, and so is the sun. A rudimentary consciousness contained in matter and living cells maintains the life in the body. He suggests that a higher consciousness, the human psyche, inhabits that body most of the time but is also independent of it.

A somewhat different approach is offered by theoretical physicist Amit Goswami, in his *The Self-Aware Universe* and in the film *What the BLEEP Do We Know!?* Goswami suggests that it is not the "wavicles" or particles that demonstrate intelligence, but the very field out of which they emerge and of which they are, necessarily, a part. Drawing on Hindu Vedic literature for descriptive language, Goswami uses the image of "Indra's Net" to describe the field of consciousness that, he suggests, is the underlying framework for all existence and is exhibited throughout space and time.

In all these quantum-theoretical approaches, two fundamental understandings are consistent, based on the experimental evidence.

- First, the fundamental units of the universe exhibit the fundamental quality of intelligence: they choose which form they will take, based on the structure of the system in which they are generated, including the thought processes of those observing the process.

- Second, all of these fundamental units of matter and energy exhibit a characteristic called nonlocality, so whenever any one of these "wavicles" is connected with another one, it will always, instantaneously, respond as if it were still connected — no matter how far apart they are in space and time.

And, as we stated earlier in this text, the wave form of energy is not limited to one point but extends throughout all space and time, all at once, overlapping with all other wave forms in complex resonating patterns.

These two characteristics, intelligence and nonlocality, pervade all of matter and energy in all its forms, and their ubiquitous presence means that, literally, no action can occur without a parallel response, elsewhere in the universe. Quantum mechanics demonstrates, then, that intelligence is truly omnipresent and that every thought or action is instantaneously felt, everywhere.

When we realize that no one is an isolated individual, that who we are is a function of the relationships in which we participate, that we are all connected through a remarkably complex system of interacting energy fields, and that it's impossible to "do just one thing," or act in isolation, we realize that to heal any one person of any one condition, including ourselves, is to increase the likelihood of healing for all others who have that condition, as well. And the reverse. The patterns of resonance work instantly, everywhere.

Global Consciousness

One of the most remarkable graphs ever produced was published on the internet by the Global Consciousness Project, housed at Princeton University, in September of 2001 (the website is http://noosphere.princeton.edu)

Generated by a computer, this graph integrates reports from thirty computers around the world, connected through the internet. These computers do two things: they generate random lists of numbers and they report back to the central computer the numbers that are generated.

Normally, the report looks like a small, squiggly line, moving back and forth across zero. What made this particular graph so amazing, however, was that on a particular date—September 11, 2001—the line spiked off the page.

As the Twin Towers collapsed in Manhattan, the numbers generated by computers all over the world were far from random. Even more amazing, the line had actually begun to vary several days before that date and continued to spike at lower levels for the next couple of days, dipping well below zero during the worldwide "three minutes of silence" at noon on Friday, the 14th.

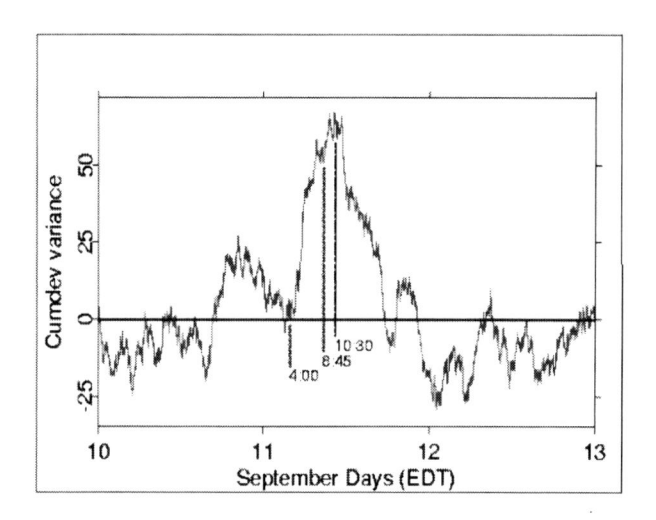

What happened here?

Random number generators (RNGs) produce series of one & zeroes that usually have no pattern. The Consciousness Project was developed to test the hypothesis that, since one person can affect the output of an RNG by focusing their intention, would a community or the whole of humanity be able to do so?

On 9/11, the answer came back an unequivocal "Yes." When people have strong thoughts or feelings, they change the pattern of 1s and 0s generated by a computer. That is, they affect the material world in measurable ways. Second, it tells us that, even before we are aware of an event, our emotions and thoughts are affected by it. Finally, it makes it clear, if it wasn't before, that, truly, nothing happens in isolation—all that we think, say, and do affects the whole world.

Since that date, the Princeton group has greatly expanded the number of computers in the network and have shown remarkable results for many events, ranging from earthquakes and tidal waves to Wold Cup play offs. Again and again demonstrating that when large numbers of people focus their intention on something or someone, they affect the material world around them.

Prayer, Meditation, and the Maharishi Effect

Most of us have been taught that prayer is a process of asking an all-powerful divinity to give us something or make something different for us. Some of us have been taught a variation on this, based on a quote from Jesus in the New Testament: "Pray, believing you have received." Some of us have learned that prayer is an ongoing communication with inner divinity, in which we express appreciation, gratitude, and praise, and through which we receive insights and deeper understandings and a peace of mind that quickly shows up in our surroundings.

Mystics from many spiritual traditions have emphasized this latter form of prayer, recognizing that through the ongoing communication with inner divinity (the Oversoul. Christ within, Goddess, Spirit guides,Buddha-nature, and other terms have been used, depending on the culture), one's sense of isolation begins to dissolve and one begins to identify with the union developed through the interaction. Their resulting ecstatic experiences and visible joy have encouraged others to do the same. From Catholic saints to Hindu gurus, from dancing "witches" to "whirling dervishes," the mystical experience of direct communion with divinity becomes a visible radiance in the person experiencing it—inviting others to do likewise.

Prayer, however, is not the words spoken, nor even the process used. Prayer is best understood as the state of consciousness that results from these activities.[243] As metaphysicians across ages and cultures have taught, it's achieving that state of consciousness that leads to results—not the grace or whim of a divine being "out there".

Meditation is in many ways like prayer. It requires turning one's thoughts away from normal life. It sets the mind at peace. It allows for greater and deeper awareness. In some ways, meditation could be considered nontheistic prayer, in which union with universal dimensions, rather than a specific divinity, is the intention.

Healing the Person, Healing the Planet

According to the model we've laid out in these pages, the energy fields that compose a human being are fully and harmoniously interacting with all other energy fields in a resonating pattern all the time. Meditation and deep prayer allow us to experience that. This means that when we pray or meditate, we're entering a harmonious state of consciousness that encourages harmony both in our own energy fields and with the fields around us.

The most harmonious state of consciousness (which can be called the state of Grace or, in Sanskrit, *satchitananda*, "love-bliss consciousness") is when we feel total union with the universe or divinity. And, whatever we are holding in our intention while in this state, whatever we intend for ourselves or others, becomes part of this harmoniously resonating pattern—within and around us. This is particularly so when someone understands and intends that the experience is with and for all.

Two of the methods offered in these pages are explicitly designed to generate this state: Transformative Compassionate Breathing and Releasing the Past. Both of them require the practitioner to let go of whatever situation or suffering that has been the focus of their attention and generate positive energy toward another and oneself. As they release the old way of being (which is the original meaning of the word sacrifice—from the Latin, "sacred-making") and compassionately step into a new relationship with self and others, they restore harmonious function within the energy body, create new resonant harmonies with other energy fields, and, in the process, open the flow between the mind-body and the other-dimensional bodies that the Buddhists call the *trikaya*.

Transcendental Meditation has been used and demonstrated statistically to be effective for reducing violence in cities and regions where a significant number (at least 1%) of the population is using the TM technique consistently.[244] This phenomenon has been labeled "the Maharishi Effect," after Maharishi Mahesh Yogi, the teacher who introduced this method to the U.S. It's simply demonstratng that when enough minds are in a harmoniously connected state, the field of the whole is more harmonious—just as when enough minds are focused, the random number generators change.

Other traditions have their own methods for achieving the same result. The "Shaman's Journey" of most indigenous peoples, "entering the Dreamtime" among Australian indigenous people, "Spell-Casting" among the Celtic Wiccans, and the "Rain Dance" of the Navajo and Hopi are a few of humanity's time-tested transpersonal transformational methods, along with many of the methods of *kriya yoga* and Vajrayana Buddhism. In each of these practices, the individual recognizes interconnectedness with the whole by going within and finding it, then experiences a shift in the self and the surrounding environment.

Whatever words are said, whatever practices or rituals are used, the goal is to achieve that state of awareness in which all is harmony, within and throughout. So it is that the world is transformed.

༄

Advancing Medical Options and Medical Science

In *Timeless Healing: Optimal Medicine, Optimal Health*, Herbert Benson reintroduces self-empowered healing into Western medicine, based on what he calls "wellness rememberd." He explains that such care will result in enormous cost savings in virtually all cases, and explains how

> ...medicine can make practical changes using wellness remembered across the board and reserving medications and procedures for those instances when they're needed and can be effective... that the medicine of the future be like a three-legged stool, balanced and supported by these three components: self-care, medications, and procedures.[245]

The emergence of such a development in the medical paradigm will depend on several factors coming together:

- an increasing respect for and insistence on noninvasive methods of mind-body science, such as meditation
- a willingness to inform the public about the healing potential of such methods
- the development of far-reaching education programs in self-care methods, such as meditation, throughout all levels of public and private education
- the establishment of authoritative training programs in self-care methods within the medical training institutions, including nursing schools, hospital administration programs, and the various training programs for doctors.

As a species we have a great need for healthcare alternatives that truly empower and enhance the wellbeing of the individual. And, at this point in history, we have the methods. The human treasure chest of effective, noninvasive meditation methods is full and accessible. This benign science can be used in most areas of healthcare, extending the kinds of care available, and lowering the cost of care. It is in every way a healthier kind of care than invasive medicine, and it may be more powerful.

In 2007 the National Institutes of Health sponsored a survey on healthcare choices that yielded remarkable results. Based on data collected from the 2007 National Health Interview (NHI) Survey,

- more than 6.3 million Americans, or 3%, use mind-body therapies because they were referred to them by their doctors.
- another 35 million or so Americans, the team estimates, have been self-referred to mind-body therapies.
- nearly 40 percent of Americans use or have used CAM treatments, and 75% of these involve mind-body therapies.
- most commonly used CAM treatments include the use of natural products, followed by deep breathing, meditation, and chiropractic treatments.
- The fastest growing CAM therapies between 2002 and 2007 include deep breathing, meditation, massage, and yoga.[246]

Yet, even now, after so much proven benefit, little progress has been made. The evolution of the species continues to be adversely affected by the widespread use of drugs, anesthesia, and surgery. The institutionalization of birth and death worldwide has become a significant sector of the world economy—that part of the system that has been called the "healthcare industry." As a result, the quality of life in birth and death is generally reduced or obstructed —and is much lower in the U.S. than many other countries.

The industrial nature of healthcare is perhaps most evident in the production and distribution of pharmaceuticals. Corporations with powerful lobbyists in Washington have shown a marked tendency to repress the establishment of medical alternatives to drugs, and have made an equally aggressive effort to encourage the use of pharmaceutical agents—through federal agency support and increased access to worldwide resources, media, and advertising. Recent scandals in the Food and Drug Administration simply highlight imbalances in a system that no longer works to protect consumers, but rather promotes corporate interests.

Another aspect of the "healthcare industry" that tends to repress nonconventional methods is the role of the insurers. Again, large corporations with significant lobbying power work in Washington and in state legislatures to ensure that their preferred methods and procedures are supported so they may maximize stockholder returns.

So, although cost reductions through mind-body medicine have been demonstrated repeatedly, the powers-that-be continue to limit access to proven methods of self-care. They see that they can't make money from its use.

Still, in spite of these deterrents, more and more people continue to learn about and choose Era II and Era III alternatives, and the body of research continues to grow—to the point where the potential of such techniques has captured the attention of the media and the medical training institutions. These noninvasive alternatives have also captured the interest of the new generation, which feels cheated and deprived of their right to a clean and healthy environment and body.

More, the passivity cultivated by a disempowering medical system of treatments by authority figures is unhealthy. The doctor's prescriptions are too often determined by corporate greed. The system often deprives people of their inalienable right to choose for themselves. Almost no one is told by medical doctors that noninvasive methods that restore health balance have been proved to be far more effective in the long run than conventional medicine's interventions that simply minimize symptoms. Era II and Era III methods restore and increase health.

The research is conclusive: meditation practices are healing and empowering. When we meditate, we help heal and empower ourselves; we tap the genius of self-care, and we radiate wellbeing into the world.

What the world needs is more and better healthcare and medical options, like teaching women about the noninvasive options in advanced natural childbirth; like offering an approach to Alzheimer's care and care for the comatose that reaches the inner awareness; like giving dying people and their loved ones a hopeful, healing process as they transition out of their bodies.

We can be certain that powerful noninvasive healthcare options are available, and education concerning this can be the basis for reform. Harvard has been warning that the medical establishment could be on the verge of collapse from malpractice lawsuits and bad economics, and when it does, self-care and mind-body medicine will be ready to help build a better medical paradigm.

Let's finish this book with a clear statement of intent. Realizing that intention is a powerful resource at our disposal, let's intend to benefit all humanity—past, present, and future. Let's intend that consciousness-transforming healing methods be offered to all people:

> May we all experience the evolutionary benefits of such practices.
>
> May we establish a timeless field of health and well-being everywhere on Earth.
>
> May self-care become everyone's experience as well as their right.
>
> May we all know self-care as planetary care.

ಌ

Appendix A:

The Light Nature of the Energy Body According to Vajrayana Buddhism

Robert Bruce Newman

We have attempted to offer an integrated model of the human body that takes into account some of the profound and comprehensive knowledge from the fields of Chinese medicine and yoga, Ayurvedic medicine, and Hindu yoga, as well as Tibetan medicine and Vajrayana Buddhist meditation science. But very little of the knowledge of the energy body in those traditions has been published. We have mentioned four kinds of *chi* functioning in the body according to Chinese medicine, and five kinds of *prana* functioning in the body according to the Hindu science of breathing. That is helpful in terms of inspiring a greater respect for the body and its subtle systems and for encouraging people to learn more about the real nature of the human body's functions and potential. But it is insufficient.

Now, though, having completed many years of study of Vajrayana Buddhist meditation science it's possible to present previously unpublished information on the nature of the energy body. This information has been confirmed through centuries of work by Tibetan meditation masters and doctors. Our hope is that medical science will progressively see more and more dimensions of life in the human body, and see the human body as the inconceivably great form of potential that it is. To that end an explanation of a complex body of energy channels (Tibetan: *tsa*) in which ten kinds of *prana* (Tibetan: *lung*) function, governed by light-bearing sexual essence (Tibetan: *thiglé*), is summarized below.

Lung

Like *chi* and *prana*, the term *lung* is often translated as "air" or "wind." *Lung* originates in the primal field of the Dharmakaya as unconditioned life force energy. That *lung* tends to differentiate into two primal luminosities, red and white, that separate out of the clear light of the Dharmakaya. In a powerful conjunction of forces at the moment of human conception, awareness, integral to the red and white luminosities, enters the union of the egg and sperm.

Ten kinds of *lung* form in the first moment of body formation. Immediately three forces act together. Light-bearing cellular units of the "mother seed essence" and the "father seed essence" retain their identities as the essence of the egg and sperm and separate out in magnetic polar connection, forming the basis of the central energy channel (CEC). The white, father seed essence is the brilliant point source (*thigle,* seed syllable) of the crown chakra. The red, mother seed essence is the brilliant seed syllable of the navel chakra. These are the basis of the *thigle* of the new body. Simultaneously, in the moment when the ten *lungs* form, a total of twelve major energy channels are formed and then flow in the channels. From this powerful first moment *tsa, lung,* and *thigle* are inseparable. Together, they hold the light basis of the human potential.

There are five principal lung movements and five subtle vital energies that derive from those movements. The five major *lungs* can be thought of as energy currents in the body. They are:

- lung holding the life force
- lung all-pervading throughout the body
- lung preventing deterioration (holding heat)
- upward-moving lung (includes digestion)
- downward-moving lung (includes elimination)

All five major lungs are held separately in the CEC. In the normal flow of *lung* through the channels, the language basis of consciousness is formed. When they are not separated, when they "push into one another," it causes an imbalance of pressures and disturbs the mind-body. The quality and interaction of the energies and *thigle* of the body affect the quality of the flow of the *lungs* in the *tsa* and movements in the mind-body.

Tsa

The *tsa* react as the *lungs* in the body react. They are not on their own, but interdependent with *lung* and its functions. Yet the major *tsa* have a fixed form that reflects the pattern of the universe. The infinite external universe is represented in the twelve main *tsa* that form at our conception. Those *tsa* reflect completely the spacelike quality of our awareness, an essential basis of the wisdom of our Buddha-nature. Eventually 72,000 main *tsa*, and related subtle *tsa*, come into form. The channels of our body are modified according to our projections of the external universe. Our habitual patterning limits the potential of energy channel functioning and results in blockages in the system. Our most subtle channels are always changing according to the activities of our mind. The largest channels, such as the CEC, are fixed in form and are integral to the body's universal functioning.

There are three main or central channels, the CEC and its two "side channels." The CEC is the trikaya. The "secret" nature of that and the secret nature of the channel systems must be realized by meditation practice. The blockages in the channels limiting the potential of energy body functioning can be released by meditation practices such as Vase Breathing or by sexual union practice.

Thigle

Thigle is a physical substance, the body's sexual essence. It governs the quality of consciousness and being in the human body. *Thigle* is considered by the Vajrayana teachers to be the most precious substance in the human body. The wanton disregard for sexual substances through widespread mindless ejaculation in both sexual engagement with partners and in masturbation is a sign of the general loss of evolutionary quality throughout the species. However, whenever people respect the male and female sexual essences and see them as sacred substances, the health and potential of the human body are safeguarded.

Vajrayana masters, such as the Dalai Lama, consider the millions of individual *thigle* to be individual buddhas. They see the waste of *thigle* to be the murder of millions of buddhas and the waste of the light potential of the human form. They also see that *thigle* may be used as sacred medicine by tantric couples.

In the vision of the Vajrayana meditation masters, *thigle* is produced from the finest essence of the digestion of food. That essence in turn is evolved into blood. The blood is filtered (distilled) into the "pure blood of the heart." This creation of blood is seen to take place in the bone marrow, which is in accord with the knowledge of Western science. However, the blood in the bone marrow, in its highest evolution, is transformed into *thigle*.

Thigle can penetrate bone and unify, in the male, with the seminal fluid in the testes. This is not known to Western science. In women the *thigle* remains closely associated with blood and is called *rhakta*. *Rhakta* is also released in orgasm, but in a much finer form and more as a whole-body emission. In the sexual union of Vajrayana practitioners, orgasm is often withheld. Thus *thigle* is contained, and the light essence of the *thigle* is used to turn awareness to the clear light nature of inherent *rigpa*, luminous clarity. If the *thigle* is released in sexual practice, its light nature is known and it is typically reabsorbed, except for some that is given to the partner as sacred substance to be used for healing or evolution.

The greatest triumph of the species, the ability to transform one's body into light (Rainbow Body; *Ja Lu*, in Tibetan), at death or earlier in life, is the result of this knowledge of the light basis of *thigle*.

Appendix B

The Issue of Will in Western Culture

Ruth L Miller

Many times in this book we've described or encouraged the use of focused intention as part of the healing process. On the surface this seems straightforward enough: if we are to accomplish anything we must first intend it.

Western culture, however, is confused on the subject of the source and basis for illness and other life circumstances. Is it an individual's will that determines his or her experience? Is it fate? Or does God have some plan for each individual that includes the particular situation we're in? In short, many people wonder, is any particular outcome God's will or the individual's?

Most of us don't give much thought to the issue until we're confronted with a situation that seems beyond our control. In the face of a terminal diagnosis, or even a business failure or pregnancy, we're inclined to say that a power beyond ourselves must be responsible. And, as we wrestle with the situation and our feelings, Christians, in particular, may find themselves saying, as Jesus the Nazarene is reported to have said, "Not my will but Thine!"—often while secretly wishing their own wish or desire would be fulfilled.

Given that most processes addressing the condition of the mind-body are strongly affected by the beliefs held by the individual, this confusion can have a marked effect on the outcome. The evidence shows that, to the extent that people hold conflicting beliefs about a situation, they will have mixed outcomes. And as the research we described earlier in this book indicates, if someone's belief in a procedure is mixed with doubt, that procedure's effectiveness is reduced.

Fortunately for believers, both the Hebrew and Christian Bibles, as well as the Qur'an, offer a powerful set of answers to the problem in the form of descriptions of God's eternal will for humanity. In fact, in many ways it's been made clear that, even though someone's actions may lead to consequences that are unpleasant, "It is God's good pleasure to give you the kingdom" [Luke 12: 32].

In the Hebrew Bible Jeremiah [29:11] says:

> 'For I know the plans that I have for you,' declares the LORD, 'plans for welfare and not for calamity, to give you a future and a hope.'

And Psalm 37:4: "Delight in the Lord and He will give you the desires of your heart."

The Christian New Testament says, in Matthew:

> What do you think? If a man has a hundred sheep, and one of them has gone astray, does he not leave the ninety-nine on the mountains and go in search of the one that went astray? And if he finds it, truly, I say to you, he rejoices over it more than over the ninety-nine that never went astray. So it is the will of my Father who is in heaven that not one of these little ones should perish. [18:11-14]

The Qur'an, too, is quite clear on the subject:

> Those who wish to receive their reward in this world will receive it, and those who wish to receive their reward in the world to come will also receive it. And We will undoubtedly reward those who serve Us with gratitude. [3:145]

In short, the various Western scriptures declare without doubt that the Will of God (whatever name is used to describe divinity) is the fulfillment of each person's heart's desires and the wellbeing of each soul.

So, what are people to do when faced with a calamity? Surely it isn't to say "it must be God's will!" Rather, it's to be very clear about what their desires are and have been!

When people come up against circumstances that seem beyond control and intolerable, it's time to be very clear. Everyone needs to ask themselves: What have we been focusing on? What have we been "sort of" wishing for? What have we been "jokingly" declaring we'd rather life were like? As many spiritual teachers have said over the course of history: in all our jokes and disparaging remarks, we've actually asked for something that is taking the form of this apparently unhappy circumstance.

Appendix B

Summarizing what we've learned, then, the Western sacred texts say that the Will of God for all humanity is that we experience health, comfort, meaningful self-expression, prosperity, and loving relationships. And it's only when one's combined heart and mind—one's total consciousness—is clearly focused on universal wellbeing, experiencing the "bliss consciousness" of *rigpa*, which can also be called "delighting in the LORD", that anyone can count on experiencing those things.

And this is what the methods we offer here can provide.

☙

Appendix C

The Material Science of the Light Body

Ruth L. Miller

During the late 1980s and early 1990s, a new understanding of the nature of matter was emerging. Previous understandings assumed that the coherent light we call a laser could only be generated with complex equipment using significant amounts of energy. Yet, in the biological journals, people were reporting photon emissions and beams of light within and between cells. Danah Zohar says,

> ...in living systems photons are *very* much more (exponentially more) bunched together, literally "squashed" into a coherent Bose-Einstein condensate... In the process of photon bunching we see the primitive antecedent of the coherence that becomes life, but on its own it is timeless—it has no sense of direction.[247]

She points out that photons are a form of boson, explaining, "Bosons are, essentially, 'particles of relationship' ... they bind together the material world".[248]

> ...ultimately we can trace our consciousness to its roots in the special kind of relationship that exists wherever two bosons meet, to their propensity to bind together, to overlap, and to share an identity. It is this propensity that makes possible the much more coherent ordering of more complex quantum systems (those found in life and human consciousness)—where millions of bosons overlap and share an identity, behaving as one large boson....[249]

"One large boson" is technically called a Bose-Einstein condensate, in which

> the many parts that go to make up an ordered system not only *behave* as a whole, they *become* whole; their identities merge or overlap in such a way that they lose their individuality entirely.[250]

Superconductors are a form of Bose-Einstein condensate. Laser beams are another. Herbert Frölich, of Liverpool University, has demonstrated that pumping energy into a system of vibrating, electrically charged molecules causes the molecules to vibrate in unison, pulling themselves into a Bose-Einstein condensate—even in living tissue. More, these vibrating molecules emit electromagnetic waves, or light.[251]

Fritz Popp has called the weak "glow" emitted by living cells, "coherent biophotons" and he, along with other scientists working in other countries have seen evidence of such "biophoton emissions" within and around the DNA molecule.[252]

Previous understandings also assumed that the core unit of matter, the atom, is extremely stable and requires great quantities of energy to be "split" or otherwise disrupted. These understandings worked very well for most experiences, but there were an increasing number of observations that didn't conform.

The data came in bit by bit, in individual research reports and letters to the various journals of physics. Some atoms, it seems, are "deformed" when separated from other atoms. They aren't spherical or even egg-shaped, but may be extended to the point of looking like a banana. These atoms can be found in the "rare earths" and other elements in the center section of the periodic table, including platinum, iridium, gold, and rhodium. When deformed, they don't act like normal atoms. They split easily, requiring very little energy to do so.[253] They arrange themselves too far apart to share electrons, yet they act as if they were highly integrated Bose-Einstein condensates, or "superconductors".[254] Because the atoms are so far apart, they don't look or act like metal, but form a white powder. Moreover, the white powder emits "phonons," (wavicles that act like light but move at the speed of sound, 1,150 miles per second, instead of the usual light-speed constant, c, which is 186,000 miles per second). Finally, when in this state, they typically weigh only 56% of their actual mass[255] and exhibit none of their usual properties in spectrometric measurements—showing up as iron, silica, and aluminum, instead.[256]

As researchers began to understand the qualities of these metals, they used new measurement methods and found that 5% of human brain tissue consists of these metals in this form—more than all the other metals ever measured in the brain.[257]

Appendix C

With these new observations, Western science begin to have an explanation for how it is that so many generations of wise people have said that we are, or have, an aura, or "body of light." If, indeed, vibrating cells emit light and if a significant amount of living tissue is composed of materials that emit low-frequency light, then all living systems are constantly emitting rays of light whose intensity and speed varies according to the vibration activity of the cells and the amount of "white powder" rare earth elements in the body.

We can go further, however. Since, as Zohar explains, the tendency of bosons "to overlap, and to share an identity" is the fundamental binding force of the atoms and molecules of which we are composed, and since bosons are that of which photons are made, then that which holds us together is the "light that is not light," which is one definition of the *rigpa* or *Dharmakaya*.

❦

Glossary

Alaya (Sanskrit.); *kunzhi* (Tibetan.): Literally it means the basis of all things, the basis of mind and phenomena. Also often called "storehouse consciousness," the basis of all karmic tendencies.

Allopathic medicine: Healing approaches that assume disease and illness are caused by elements outside of the body that have invaded it and must be killed or removed to restore health. Usually used in contrast to homeopathic or naturopathic medicine, which tend to rely on and support the body's internal healing resources.

Ati yoga (Skt.); *Dzogchen* (Tib.): Natural Great Perfection; innate primordial wisdom, free of path or method. Mind-made views and meditations are shattered by free awareness. Disturbing emotions are liberated without any need for reform or remedy. This instruction brings realization not produced from causes. It is instantaneous liberation in wisdom, in the power plenum of absolute space.

Audio-guidance: The use of audio recordings to guide those who listen to facilitate a shift into greater function.

Awareness (Tib. *rigpa*; Skt. *vidya*): When referring to the view of the Great Perfection, "awareness" means self-cognizing consciousness devoid of ignorance and dualistic fixation.

Bardo (Tib.); *antarabhava* (Skt.): The intermediate state. Usually refers to the period between death and the next rebirth. There are also three bardos in the present life.

Bindu (Skt.); *thigle* (Tib.): A luminous and brilliant seed syllable. May refer to the point between the eyebrows that connects with the "third eye" chakra. See thigle.

Bodhicitta (Skt.): "Awakened state of mind." Wisdom heart. (1) The aspiration to attain enlightenment for the sake of all sentient beings. (2) In the context of Dzogchen, the innate wakefulness of awakened mind; synonymous with rigpa, luminous awareness.
Buddha-nature: The potential for enlightenment or enlightened nature that is inherently present in each sentient being.

Bum Chung (Tib.): Small or Gentle Vase Breathing. It is not *Bum Chen*, Large Vase Breathing, which must be practiced under the close supervision of an accomplished master. Throughout this book the term Vase Breathing refers to Small Vase Breathing, also called "breathing on top of." It may be applied in various medical applications as an awareness-based energy body method.

Chi (*Qi*): Vital energy. There is external and internal chi. "Chi is fundamental to Chinese medical thinking, yet no one English word or phrase can adequately capture its meaning. Perhaps we can think of Chi as matter on the verge of becoming energy or energy at the point of materializing" (Kaptchuk 1983, 35).

Complementary and Alternative Medicine (CAM): The term for various medical disciplines, mostly traditional, now included in the expanded medical paradigm. Dissatisfaction with conventional medical practices has created great popular interest in and respect for CAM.

Dharmakaya (Skt.); *cho* (Tib.): The first of the three *kayas*, devoid of world but full of extremely powerful energy. It is unmanifest and is inseparable from its form bodies, the *Sambhogakaya* and the *Nirmanakaya*. It is also often used equivalent to *rigpa*.

Dzogchen (Tib.): See Ati yoga.

Empowerment (Tib. *wang*): The conferring of power or authorization to practice the Vajrayana teachings.

Energy medicine: Medical practices wherein the body is seen to be a body of energy systems and fields; practices of seeing and modifying those fields therapeutically constitutes diagnosis and treatment. Acupuncture, acupressure, bodywork, healing touch, and conscious breathing are each a kind of energy medicine.

Fine breathing: Deep breathing that intentionally absorbs vital energy from the air as well as accessing optimal oxygenation.

Guru Rinpoche (Tib.): "Precious Master," the "Second Buddha" who established Vajrayana Buddhism in Tibet in the ninth century. He is also known as Padmasambhava. His compassionate omniscience is with us today in his terma (concealed treasures) in Vajrayana practice. His methods may enlighten the present and free the future.

Habitual tendencies: Inclinations imprinted in the alaya consciousness that can be released by the experience of *rigpa*.

Hara (Jap.): The vital center; focal point of Zen meditation, comparable to and perhaps the same as the *Tan Tien* in Chinese *Tai Chi* meditation and the Life Vase (*Tse Bum*) in Tibetan Vajrayana meditation. It is a receiver for energies breathed into it, for greater function and increase of life force.

Kaya (Skt.); *Ku* (Tib.): Body—simultaneously *Dharmakaya* (unmanifest body), body of light (*Sambhogakaya*), and flesh and blood in form (*Nirmanakaya*).

Luminosity (Tib. *orsel*): Literally "free from the darkness of unknowing and endowed with the ability to cognize." The two aspects are empty luminosity, like clear open sky, and manifest luminosity, such as five rays of color, images, brilliant spheres of *thigle*. Luminosity is the uncompounded nature present throughout all the world.

Mantra (Skt.): Combinations of seed sound syllables, brilliant *bindu*, radiating healing light from the sound. Almost all mantras start with the radiant bindu OM, the crown chakra, purifying body into sacred body. Mantra also protects the mind. It gives practitioners enlightened sound that resonates healing in the body channels during recitation.

Meditation: A practice that enables people to experience greater levels of awareness and health by shifting consciousness to its essential state, normally blocked by the mind in its undisciplined activity.

Meditation science: The scientific knowledge behind meditation methods from different traditions, with understanding of the short- and long-term effects of the application of those methods. These methods have been tested and proved through centuries of disciplined use, yielding repeatable results in accordance with the scientific method.

Mind-body medicine: A major development in the history of medicine, expanding the medical paradigm in the West since the 1970s, in which meditation and other interventions using the mind enable the body to improve its function. Called self-care in this text, it's seen as the heart of a new medical paradigm.

Mindfulness-Based Stress Reduction (MBSR): The renowned mindbody medicine clinic at the University of Massachusetts Medical Center. Established in 1979, it has trained more than 18,000 people in medicine/meditation methods and has been the model for hundreds of such programs established in the United States, Canada, and Europe.

Nadi (Skt.); *tsa* (Tib.): Energy channel. For full description of the energy channels and their function in accord with *lung* and *thigle*, see the Appendix.

Nectar medicine (Tib. *dutsie*; Skt. *amrita*: the nectar of immortality): A consecrated combination of sacred herbs and blessed substances, energetically endowed with healing power.

Nirmanakaya (Skt.); *tulku* (Tib.): Emanation body. The form kaya of the three kayas. Form of magical apparition. The aspect of enlightenment that can be perceived by ordinary beings.

Optimal breathing: A practice, such as Womb Breathing, in which vital energy from the air and oxygen are breathed.

Padmasambhava: See Guru Rinpoche.

Paradigm: A pattern, example, or model. A concept accepted by most people in an intellectual community that informs and determines their perceptions and actions.

Paradigm shift: A change in the way individuals or cultures interpret phenomena, a sense of having new eyes or new knowing, leading to new ways of behaving.

Pointing-out instruction (Tib. *mengagde*): The direct instruction given by the teacher so that the disciple recognizes the nature of mind.

Prana (Skt.); *lung* (Tib.): A subtle but powerful life energy pervading all matter; universal life force. Energy currents in the body and in the external universal field. Probably the same as *chi*. Western science refers to it as universal energy. It can be breathed and utilized, as in the practice of Vase Breathing.

Reiki (Jap.): A form of natural healing in which universal life force energy flows through the practitioner to the receiver to augment and enhance the natural healing ability inherent in the human body. Reiki balances, strengthens, and harmonizes the connection between body, mind, and spirit, promoting a sense of wellbeing on all levels, for both practitioner and patient.

Sambhogakaya (Skt.); *Long Ku* (Tib.): Between the unmanifest body of the *Dharmakaya* and the manifest body of the *Nirmanakaya* is the semi-manifest body of the *Sambhogakaya*. Referred to as body of bliss, body of communication, it is practiced and experienced as a sacred body of light radiating effectively into the world.

Shamatha (Skt.): Calm Abiding. A meditation practice for calming down and staying calm in order to rest free of the disturbances of the mind. Various concentration techniques are used. The most common is following the breath.

Slow breathing: Deep breathing becomes slow breathing, healthier breathing, using minimal energy. Ancient wisdom says that each life has a certain number of breaths to live, and intentionally slowed breathing brings long life.

Subtle body: Inner body, or energy body. Sometimes called astral, mental, and causal bodies, these bodies have been seen to be operating at successively higher frequencies than the physical body. In Buddhist practice the subtle bodies are the *Dharmakaya* and *Sambhogakaya*. They are engaged, activated, and utilized by evolutionary work. Medicine today is more accepting of the presence of an energy body in the physical body, in which subtle body functions are integral to physical functions.

Superknowledge (Skt. *Abhijna*): Powers that naturally arise from meditation, such as those that irreversibly manifested in Shakyamuni Buddha in his enlightenment, and in those who have followed in his path: divine sight; divine hearing; recollection of former lives; cognition of the minds of others; capacity for performing miracles; and in the case of accomplished practitioners, the cognition of the exhaustion of habitual patterns and obscurations.

Tan Tien (Chinese): Focal point for *Tai Chi* meditation, situated in the navel center. The *Tan Tien* is similar to the Life Vase or *Hara*, and may be the same.

Tantra (Skt.): Continuity. The Vajrayana teachings given by the Buddha in his *Sambhogakaya* form. The innate Buddha-nature, which is known as the "tantra of the expressed meaning" in the extraordinary tantric scriptures also known as the "tantra of the expressing words." Can also refer to the resultant teachings of the Vajrayana as a whole.

Terma (Tib.): Treasure. Transmission through concealed treasures, hidden mainly by Guru Rinpoche and Yeshe Tsogyal, to be revealed at the right time by a terton, a treasure revealer, for the benefit of all.

Thigle (Tib.); *bindu* (Skt.): Aluminous and radiant seed syllable found in the center of each of the chakras; also, sperm. See Appendix A for detail of function in the energy body.

Trikaya (Skt.): the combination of *Dharmakaya, Sambhogakaya*, and *Nirmanakaya*. The three *kayas* as ground are essence, nature, and expression; as path they are bliss, clarity, and nonthought; and as fruition they are the three *kayas* of Buddhahood.

Vajra (Skt.); *dorje* (Tib.): "Diamond," "king of stones." As an adjective it means "indestructible," "invincible," or "firm." The ultimate *vajra* is emptiness, complete openness; the conventionally understood *vajra* is a ritual implement, mostly cast metal.

Vajrayana: The Diamond Vehicle; the Buddhism of Tibet; the ultimate stage of the development of the Buddha's teachings. Based on the vow of compassionate service to all life, Vajrayana Buddhism is known for its variety of profound methods.

Vase Breathing: This practice, a treasure of ancient wisdom, is characterized by breathing vital essence from the air down into the Life Vase, *Tse Bum*, in the navel center, which feeds the energy up into the central psychic channel for greater function.

Vipashyana (Skt.) (also written Vipassana): Clear or wider seeing; panoramic awareness; extraordinary insight; "Wisdom Mind" arising from *Shamatha* practice. Also a psychological basis of Vase Breathing.

Visualization: A concentration method in which the mind is focused on an image or a situation with as much detail as possible to maximize the intensity of the experience. In healing visualizations, the whole body, a specific body system, or body process is envisioned purposefully, to alter the body's biology beneficially. To be most successful visualization should be based on calming meditation. In practices such as Vase Breathing, the energy body and its systems are visualized to access their potential.

Yoga: Literally "union." Originally a general category for various kinds of meditation practice, today in the West, the term *yoga* usually refers to *hatha yoga*, stretching and breathing exercises, which can be beneficial in maintaining muscle tone and stamina. At least seven other *yogas* are practiced in Hindu traditions. Tibetan *yoga* practice is based on Vase Breathing and a progressive development of the realization and utilization of the potential of the energy body.

ೞ

Concise Bibliography of Vajrayana Literature in English

Chagdud Tulku. Gates to Buddhist Practice. Junction City, CA: Padma Publishing, 2001.

Chang, G. C. C. The Six Yogas of Naropa. Ithaca, NY: Snow Lion Publications, 1963.

Clifford, Terry. Tibetan Buddhist Medicine and Psychiatry: The Diamond Healing. New York: Samuel Weiser, Inc., 1984.

Dalai Lama. A Flash of Lightning in the Dark of Night. Boston: Shambhala Publications, 1994.

———. Sleeping, Dreaming, and Dying. Boston: Wisdom Publications, 1997.

Dilgo Khyentse. The Heart Treasure of the Enlightened Ones. Boston: Shambhala Publications, 1992.

Dowman, Keith. Sky Dancer: The Secret Life and Songs of the Lady Yeshe Tsogyal. London: Routledge & Kegan Paul, 1984.

Dudjom Rinpoche. Counsels from My Heart. Boston: Shambhala Publications, 2001.

———. The Nyingma School of Tibetan Buddhism. London: Wisdom Publications, 1991.

Fremantle, Francesca. Luminous Emptiness. Boston: Shambhala Publications, 2001.

——— and Chogyam Trungpa. The Tibetan Book of the Dead. Berkeley, CA: Shambhala Publications, 1975.

Gyatrul Rinpoche. Ancient Wisdom. Ithaca, NY: Snow Lion Publications, 1993.

Manjusrimitra. Primordial Experience. Boston: Shambhala Publications, 1987.

Padmasambhava. Dakini Teachings. Boston: Shambhala Publications, 1990.

———. Natural Liberation. Boston: Wisdom Publications, 1998. 340

Reynolds, John. The Golden Letters. Ithaca, NY: Snow Lion Publications, 1996.

———. Self-Liberation Through Seeing with Naked Awareness. Barrytown, NY: Station Hill Press, 1989.

Sogyal Rinpoche. The Tibetan Book of Living and Dying. New York: HarperCollins, 1994.

Thinley Norbu Rinpoche. White Sail. Boston: Shambhala Publications, 1992.

Trungpa, Chogyam. The Collected Works. Boston: Shambhala Publications, 2004.

Tsele Natsok Rangdrol. The Mirror of Mindfulness. Boston: Shambhala Publications, 1989.

Tulku Thondup Rinpoche. Hidden Teachings of Tibet. London: Wisdom Publications, 1986.

———. The Practice of Dzogchen: Writings of Longchen Rabjam. Ithaca, NY: Snow Lion Publications, 1989.

———. The Tantric Tradition of the Nyingma. Marion, MA: Buddhayana,

1984.

Yeshe Tsogyal. The Lotus-Born: The Life Story of Padmasambhava.

Boston: Shambhala Publications, 1993.

End Notes

Introduction

[1] Dudjom Rinpoche, *Dudjom Tesar Ngondro*, New York: Yeshe Melong, 1984, p. 31.
[2] Sogyal Rinpoche, *The Tibetan Book of Living and Dying* San Francisco: HarperSanFrancisco, 1994, p. 256.
[3] Ibid., 255; also referred to by various Christian mystics and shamans.
[4] Herbert Benson. *Timeless Healing: Optimal Medicine, Optimal Health*. New York: Scribner, 1996, p. 22.
[5] American Medical Association. News release. April 14, 1998.
[6] Herbert Benson. *Timeless Healing: Optimal Medicine, Optimal Health*. New York: Scribner, 1996.
[7] American Medical Association, news release. April 14, 1998.
[8] Richard Grossinger, *Planet Medicine*. Berkeley, CA: North Atlantic Books, 2000 p. 538.
[9] Marilyn Ferguson,. *The Aquarian Conspiracy*. Los Angeles: Tarcher, 1980, pp. 242–3, 250.
[10] Herbert Benson,. *Timeless Healing: Optimal Medicine, Optimal Health*. New York: Scribner, 1996,

Mind-Body Medicine Comes of Age

[11] Deepak Chopra,. *Quantum Healing*. New York: Bantam, 1990, p. 70.
[12] Deepak Chopra,. *Creating Health*. Boston: Houghton-Mifflin, 1987.
[13] Schlitz, M. and T. Amorok. *Consciousness and Healing; Integral Approaches to Mind-Body Medicine*; Elsevier, St. Louis, MO: 2005.
[14] Candace Pert, *Molecules of Emotion*. New York: Touchstone, 1997.
[15] Bruce Lipton. *The Biology of Belief*. Santa Rosa, CA: Elite Books, 2005.
[16] Michael Murphy, *The Future of the Body: Explorations into the Further Evolution of Human Nature*. Los Angeles: Tarcher, 1992.
[17] Ibid., p. 544.
[18] Norman Cousins. *Anatomy of an Illness from a Patient's Perspective*. New York: Norton, 1979.
[19] Ibid. p. 132.
[20] Ibid., p. 133.
[21] Irving Kirsch,. *The Emperor's New Drugs,* 2012.
[22] Gabor Mate, *When the Body Says No; exploring the stress-disease connection*. Wiley, 2003, p.239
[23] ibid, p.231

[24] Ibid. pp 231-237
[25] www.therapeutictouchnetwork. org 1999.
[26] Wirth, D. 1990. "The Effect of Non-Contact Therapeutic Touch on the Healing of Full Thickness Dermal Wounds." Subtle Energies 1 (1990).
[27] Gregg Braden,. *The Isaiah Effect*. New York: Three Rivers Press, 2000.
[28] Michael I.Weintraub, "Qigong and Neurologic Illness." published in Alternative and Complementary Treatments in Neurologic Illness, New York: Elsevier, 2001, pp 197-220.
[29] www.thehealingtrust.org-uk. homepage
[30] Elmer Green and Alyce Green. *Beyond Biofeedback*. New York: Dell, 1977, p. 42–43.
[31] Kevin A Barrows, and Bradly P. Jacobs. "Mind-Body Medicine: An Introduction and Review of the Literature," draft, September 2001, p. 20.
[32] Michael Murphy,. *The Future of the Body: Explorations into the Further Evolution of Human Nature*. Los Angeles: Tarcher, 1992
[33] ibid
[34] G. Frank Lawlis,. *Transpersonal Medicine*. Boston: Shambhala, 1996.
[35] Jeanne Achterberg. *Imagery in Healing*. Boston: Shambhala, 1985, 123–24
[36] G. Frank Lawlis,. *Transpersonal Medicine*. Boston: Shambhala, 1996, 115.
[37] Ibid., 109
[38] Ibid., xvi-xvii
[39] www.noetic.com
[40] Thomas Kuhn,. *The Structure of Scientific Revolutions*, Chicago: University of Chicago Press, 1962.

Meditation Methods Across Cultures

[41] Willard Johnson,. *Riding the Ox Home: A History of Mdeitation from Shamanism to Science*, 2008
[42] Mircea Eliade, *Shamanism: Archaic Techniques of Ecstasy*, 1966.
[43] New Testament, Book of Acts.
[44] General Bernardo Rosini of the United Air Command: "Each time that the pilots returned from their missions,they spoke of this Friar that appeared in the sky and diverted their airplanes, making them turn back. "…he Commanding General of USAF general Nathan F. Twining who happened to be in Bari, and decided to pilot himself a squadron of bombers to destroy a target near San Giovanni Rotondo. Whe he and his pilots were in the vicinity of the target they saw the figure of a monk with upraised hands appear in the sky. The bombs got loose from the plains falling in open areas, and the planes made a sharp turn to return to base without the pilots intervening. Back on the ground everybody asked everybody else about the happening and wanted to know who was that friar. The General was told about Padre Pio and decided to visit him with the pilots in that squadron. The pilots Immediately recognized Padre Pio, and he told the general: "So you are the one that wanted to destroy everything." Alfonso D'Artega serving at the Air Base of Amendola reported:

"One of the pilots said:' I saw the phantom fly again.'" "Another pilot saw a figure of a monk flying as fast as the plain waving his arms. The pilots and copilots saw it. "D'Artega and a pilot went to visit Padre Pio, and the pilot recognized in Padre Pio the monk seen through the clouds.

[45] Ron Roth, *The Healing Power of Prayer,* Three Rivers Press, 1998.
[46] Parfitt 1994, 101ff.
[47] Joel Goldsmith, *A Parenthesis in Eternity,* 1962: 219
[48] Emma Hopkins,. *Esoteric Philosophy,* WiseWoman Press, 2009: p, 26 (also *Emma Curtis Hopkins' Spiritual Science,* Beyond Words/Atria, 2013.)
[49] R. L. Miller, 150 Years of Healing, the lives and teachings of America's great New Thought Leaders, Abib, 2000. Distributed by WiseWoman Press.
[50] Ernest Holmes, *The Science of Mind,* 1997 edition: 146-163
[51] Christopher Isherwood and Prabhavananda, *How To Know God, the Yoga Aphorisms of Patanjali,* 1953, 221
[52] ibid., 64–66
[53] ibid., 66
[54] ibid., 68
[55] ibid., 182ff.
[56] Paramahansa Yogananda, *Autobiography of a Yogi,* Self-Ralization Fellowship, 275ff.
[57] Deepak Chopra, *Quantum Healing,* 1990, 237.
[58] Ibid.
[59] Ibid., p. 238
[60] Ibid.
[61] Clifford, 1984 referred to in *Recognition of Pain and Distress in Laboratory Animals,* "Control of Pain" published by the Institute of Laboratory Animal Resources, 1992, 53
[62] Ibid.
[63] Because Buddhism grew out of Hinduism many Hindu terms and practices have been maintained within the Buddhist tradition—even as some Judaic practices remain in Christianity and Islam.
[64] A bibliography with reference to Tibetan history, psychology, and medicine is presented in the back of this book. We encourage people to read at least Yeshe Tsogyal's *The Lotus-Born*, her record of the life of Padmasambhava and the events that followed his arrival in Tibet.
[65] Clifford, ibid., 56
[66] ibid, 58
[67] We can offer information here because Robert was the recipient of some of those teachings and transmissions through Dudjum Rinpoche, Shenphen Dawa Rinpoche, and others.
[68] Yeshe Tsogyal, *The Lotus-Born*
[69] *Rinpoche* is a title that means "cherished" or "beloved"
[70] There are several lineages of teachings in the Tibetan Buddhist tradition. The Dalai Lama is part of the *Ganden* lineage, which encourages celibate monasticism. His meditation teacher, Dudjom Rinpoche, was part of the

Nyingma lineage, which encourages marriage and family as part of one's spiritual practice.
[71] This is the center that Robert was part of and helped to manage for some decades.
[72] Barrows and Jacobs 2001, 10
[73] Depraz, Varela, and Vermersch 2000, 1
[74] Jon Kabat-Zinn 1990, 2
[75] Depraz, Varela, and Vermersch 2000, p. 15
[76] ibid., 56–61

Meditation Research

[77] Michael Murphy, *The Future of the Body*, 1992, p. 33
[78] Michael Murphy and H. Donovan, *The Physical and Psychological Effects of Meditation* 1999, p. 39ff.
[79] Ibid., 41
[80] Ibid.
[81] Kenneth Pelletier, *Mind as Healer/Mind as Slayer*, 1975, p. 226
[82] Jon Kabat-Zinn 1990, 61
[83] Herbert Benson *Timeless Healing: Optimal Medicine, Optimal Health*. New York: Scribner 1996, 146
[84] ibid, 132
[85] Joan Borysenko, 1988: 13
[86] www.tm.org
[87] www.tm.org
[88] www.ornish.com
[89] "Time series impact assessment analysis of reduced international conflict and terrorism: Effects of large assemblies of participants in the Transcendental Meditation and TM-Sidhi programs," presented at the American Political Science Association Annual Meeting, Atlanta, Georgia, August 1989.
[90] Dean Ornish 1990
[91] www.ornish.com
[92] Michael Murphy & H. Donovan, *The Physical and Psychological Effects of Meditation* 1999, 81ff.
[93] Jon Kabat-Zinn 1990, 77–78
[94] from www.sfgate.com: www.bewellbuzz.com/wellness-buzz/meditation-for-brain/
[95] Ibid.
[96] Herbert Benson. *Timeless Healing: Optimal Medicine, Optimal Health*. New York: Scribner, 1996, 130
[97] Jon Kabat-Zinn 1990
[98] Reiter and Robinson 1995, 131
[99] Chopra 1990, 62
[100] Kenneth Pelletier, *Mind as Healer/Mind as Slayer*, 1975, p. 197)

[101] Ibid, p. 192
[102] ibid, p. 193
[103] Daniel Goleman, *Emotional Intelligence,* 1995 p. 76
[104] Herbert Benson. *Timeless Healing: Optimal Medicine, Optimal Health.* New York: Scribner, 1996, 146
[105] www.ama-assn.org
[106] Dean Ornish 1990
[107] Herbert Benson *Timeless Healing: Optimal Medicine, Optimal Health.* New York: Scribner, 1996, 128
[108] Dean Ornish, 1990
[109] Daniel Goleman, *Emotional Intelligence,* 1995
[110] ibid., 173
[111] ibid., 185
[112] Herbert Benson. *Timeless Healing: Optimal Medicine, Optimal Health.* New York: Scribner, 1996, 57
[113] Larry Pelletier 1975, 192
[114] Murphy & Donovan, *The Physical and Psychological Effects of Meditation* 1999. 45–57
[115] ibid., 50
[116] Goleman and Schwartz 1976, 456, cited in Murphy & Donovan, above.
[117] Margery, 1981b, 1983, cited in Murphy & Donovan, above
[118] Murphy and Donovan, *The Physical and Psychological Effects of Meditation* 1999, 76
[119] ibid.
[120] ibid., 77
[121] Jeanne Achterberg 1985, 196
[122] Caroline Myss, *Why People Don't Heal and How They Can* 1997, 160
[123] Daniel Goleman, *Emotional Intelligence,* 1995, 76
[124] Larry Dossey, 1992, 164
[125] One of the authors, Ruth, has direct experience of this effect, having had several caesarian-section births and some dental procedures during which the treating staff expressed amazement that her pain indicators were so low.

States of Consciousness—Emerging Understandings

[126] Charles T. Tart, *Altered States of Consciousness,* 1969, p, 4
[127] ibid, p. 2
[128] Charles T.Tart, *States of Consciousness,* 1975, 28
[129] ibid., 29
[130] ibid., 30
[131] ibid., 31
[132] Joseph Chilton Pearce, *The Crack in the Cosmic Egg,* 1971
[133] William James, *The Variety of Religious Experiences* 1978, p.401

[134] H. Ross Ashby,, *Cybenetics, An Introduction,* 1962.
[135] Gregory Bateson,, *Steps to an Ecology of Mind,* 1972.
[136] Georges Gurdjieff,, quoted in Tart, 1975, 165
[137] Itshak Bentov, *Stalking the Wild Pendulum,* 1977, p. 76
[138] Ibid., p. 90
[139] Charles T. Tart, *States of Consciousness,* 1975, 182ff.
[140] This model is consistent with the teachings of *A Course in Miracles.*
[141] Itshak Bentov, *Stalking the Wild Pendulum,* 1977, p. 90
[142] Charles T. Tart, *Altered States of Consciousness*
[143] The Hebrew word *yada* (derived from the Sanskrit), which is usually translated as "to know" and sometimes refers to sexual intercourse, suggests the same idea of "union with," rather than "understanding of," that the Tibetan word *rigpa* suggests.
[144] Ilya Prigogine, and Stenger. *Order out of Chaos,* Bantam, 1984.
[145] Dharma Singh Khalsa 2001, 55
[146] Ramacharaka, *The Hindu-Yogi Science Of Breath,* a project Gutenberg text, ch IV.
[147] Govindan 1991, 154, 156
[148] Kaptchuk 1983, 35
[149] Brennan 1990, 63
[150] Lynn McTaggart, *The Field*
[151] Bruce Lipton *Biology of Belief,* 2005.
[152] in James Oschman 2000, ix
[153] Ibid.
[154] Masaru Emoto, *Messages from Water,* Japan; and *The Hidden Messages in Water,* Beyond Words, 2005.
[155] Richard Gerber, MD,*Vibrational Medicine* ,1988, p. 121
[156] ibid. 1988, 128)
[157] R.O.Becker, & G.Seldon, *The Body Electric: Electromagnetism and the Foundation of Life.* London, William Morrow. 1989., pp82-85.
[158] Francesca Fremantle, *Luminous Emptiness,* 2001, p, 263
[159] ibid., 193
[160] ibid., 190
[161] Dharma Singh Khalsa 2001, p.131
[162] ibid., p. 23
[163] Dharma Singh Khalsa 2001, p.23
[164] See *Quantum Self* by Danah Zohar for a lively explanation.
[165] James Oschman 2000, 62
[166] Claude Swanson, *Life Force; The Scientific Basis* (2011), p.186
[167] ibid. p. 170
[168] ibid. p.467
[169] Sogyal Rinpoche 1994, 263–65
[170] Francesca Fremantle *Luminous Emptiness,* 2001, p.193
[171] Lo, Huang, and Chang 2003, 620

[172] ibid.
[173] Chang, 1963, 57–60
[174] Barbara Brennan. *Hands of Light,* 1990, p. 41.
[175] Itshak Bentov, *Stalking the Wild Pendulum* 1977, pp. 56, 76
[176] Karl Maret, in Oschman 2003, ix
[177] ibid
[178] James Oschman, *Energy Medicine: The Scientific Basis* 2000, 35–37
[179] ibid., 219
[180] Carlos Castaneda, *The Active Side of Infinity,* 1998, 70
[181] Itshak Bentov, *Stalking th Wild Pendulum,* 1977, 30
[182] Iona Miller and Richard Miller 2004
[183] Several sources on the internet report this, and Gregg Braden, a geologist and computer scientist, appears most often as the source, referring to studies in Russia.
[184] Rupert Sheldrake, *A New Science of Life* 1981
[185] Rupert Shledrake interview "The Body Field" in *The Lifing Matric* dvd.
[186] Ibid.
[187] Rupert Sheldrake, *A New Science of Life* 1981., 77
[188] ibid.,189–90
[189] Oliver W. Markley and Willis Harman, *Changing Images of Man,* Stanford Research Institute, 1975 Addison-Wesley, 1984.
[190] One of the miracles of Mother Teresa's work was that she persuaded the Roman Catholic Church to allow her to focus on tending the dying bodies of the "unsaved"—not as a means to save them, but because they were, in her eyes, the embodiment of Christ.
[191] Ruth L Miller, *150 Years of Healing, the lives & teachings of America's Great Healers* (available at www.portalcenterpress.com).
[192] Anne Kennedy Winner. *The Basic Ideas of Occult Wisdom,* 1970, p. 35.
[193] Richard Gerber, MD,*Vibrational Medicine* 1988), p. 167
[194] Rama 1979, 10, 13
[195] Amit Goswami, *The Self-Aware Universe,* 1993.
[196] Francesca Fremantle, *Luminous Emptiness*,2001, p, 178
[197] ibid.
[198] ibid., 180
[199] ibid.,75
[200] ibid., 180
[201] ibid., 185
[202] ibid., 193

A New Model of Healing

[203] Larry Dossey, endorsement of Richard Gerber's *Vibrational Medicine* 1988
[204] Miller, R.L., *150 Years of Healing; the lives and teachings of* great

American healers, Abib, Portland, OR, 1999.

New Understandings of the Body... Medicine

[205] G. Frank Lawlis, 1996, xvi
[206] ibid., 5
[207] ibid, 6
[208] Dossey 1999; Schlitz et al. 2005; Murphy 1992
[209] David Wilcock, *The Source Field Investigations*, New York, Dutton, 2011. pp 95-96.
[210] Norman Cousins 1981
[211] Larry Dossey 1993
[212] Caroyln Myss, *Anatomy of the Spirit*, p. 33
[213] Sogyal 1994, 194
[214] Carl Jung, 1961, 322
[215] Gerald Jampolsky, *Teach Only Love* and *Forgiveness*
[216] Gabor Mate, *When the Body Says No*, Wiley, 2003.

The Methods

[217] Kevin A. Barrows, and Bradly P. Jacobs. "Mind-Body Medicine: An Introduction and Review of the Literature," draft, September 2001
[218] Edmund Jacobson 1938, xii; 430
[219] ibid., 429
[220] ibid., 15
[221] ibid, 406
[222] Douglas Bernstein and Thomas Borovec, 1973.
[223] Jon Kabat-Zinn, *Full Catastrophe Living*. New York: Bantam-Doubleday, 1979, 1990
[224] MediGrace was originally founded by Robert Bruce Newman as the World Health Foundation in New York and is now located in Southern Oregon. More information can be found by searching the website: www.medigrace.org.
[225] Robert Bruce Newman, *Calm Birth*, North Atlantic Books 2005. p.36
[226] Herbert Benson. *Timeless Healing: Optimal Medicine, Optimal Health*. New York: Scribner, 1996, 164
[227] Michael Murphy, 1993, 105-6
[228] Wallace, 1970; Strobel, 1975; Pelletier, 1977
[229] Michael Murphy. *The Future of the Body: Explorations into the Further Evolution of Human Nature*. Los Angeles: Tarcher, 1992, p. 544
[230] For examples see Lawliss, *Transpersonal Medicine;* Murphy, *The Future of the Body*.
[231] Ibid. p244.
[232] Florence Scovel Shinn, *The Game of Life and How to Play It*, or Ruth

Miller's *The NEW Gave of Life and How to Play it,* Beyond Words, 2012..
[233] Sogyal, *The Tibetan Book of Living & Dying,* 1996. 187ff.
[234] ibid., 208
[235] Rachel Naomi Remen, *Kitchen Table Wisdom,* p. 300
[236] *A New Model of The Healing Process: Audioguidance* p. 154-5 in the published edition; presently on p.108.
[237] Technology Review online, Feb 8, 2012

Healing the Person; Healing the Planet

[238] Larry Dossey 1989
[239] Arnold Mindell, *Working With the Dreaming Body*.London, England. Penguin-Arkana 1984, p. 5
[240] Ibid., p. 4
[241] Ibid.
[242] Itzhak Bentov, *Stalking the Wild Pendulum,*1977, p.147–48
[243] See Ruth Miller's *Uncommon Prayer* (WiseWoman Press, 2008) for an explanation of how this works.
[244] More information about these processes may be found on the website www.tm.org and the films *The Secret* and *What the Bleep Do We Know!?*
[245] Herbert Benson, *Timeless Healing* ch 10.
[246] (http://nccam.nih.gov/news/camstats/2007/camsurvey_fs1.htm

Appendix C

[247] Danah Zohar, *The Quantum Self,* New York; William Morrow, 1990. p. 223
[248] ibid. p. 224
[249] ibid. p. 222
[250] ibid. p. 83
[251] Frolich, H. and Keyzer, F., *Modern Bioelectrochemisty,* Plenum, New York, 1986
[252] Fritz-Albert Popp, "Physical Aspects of Biophotons," *Experientia,* Vol. 44, 1988.
[253] Greiner,W., Sandulescu, A. "New Radioactivities," *Scientific American,* March, 1990
[254] *Physical Review Letters,* Vol 62 #10, March 6, 1989
[255] Puthoff, Harold E., "Everything for Nothing," *New Scientist,* July 28, 1990
[256] Hudson, D. "Alchemy: Portland Presentation," video, 1998
[257] Ibid.

General References

- Achterberg, Jeanne. Imagery in Healing. Boston: Shambhala, 1985.
- American Medical Association website: www.ama-assn.org.
- Ashby, H. Ross. An Introduction to Cybernetics. New York: Pergamon, 1964.
- Bahm, Archie. Yoga Sutras of Patanjali. Albuquerque, NM: University of New Mexico Press, 1961.
- Bailey, Alice. From Intellect to Intuition. Wheaton, IL: Quest Books, 1932, 1974.
- Barrows, Kevin A., and Bradly P. Jacobs. "Mind-Body Medicine: An Introduction and Review of the Literature," draft, September 2001.
- Bateson, Gregory. Steps to an Ecology of Mind. New York: Ballantine, 1972.
- Becker, R.O. & Seldon, G. The Body Electric: Electromagnetism and the Foundation of Life. London, William Morrow. 1989.
- Benson, Herbert. The Relaxation Response. New York: William Morrow & Co., 1975.
- ———. Timeless Healing: The Power & Biology of Belief. New York: Scribner, 1996.
- Bentov, Itzhak. Stalking the Wild Pendulum. Rochester, VT: Destiny Books, 1977.
- Bernstein, Douglas and Thomas Borkovec, Progressive Relaxation, A Manual for the Helping Professions, Research Press, June 1, 1973.
- Borysenko, Joan. Minding the Body, Mending the Mind. New York: Bantam, 1988.
- Braden, Gregg. The Isaiah Effect. New York: Three Rivers Press, 2000.
- Brennan, Barbara. Hands of Light. New York: Bantam, 1990.
- Capra, Fritjof. The Tao of Physics. New York: Bantam, 1984.
- Castaneda, Carlos. The Active Side of Infinity. Toronto: HarperCollins Canada, 1998.
- Chang, G. C. C. Six Yogas of Naropa. Ithaca, NY: Snow Lion, 1963.
- Chopra, Deepak. Boundless Energy. New York: Harmony Books, 1995.
- ———. Quantum Healing. New York: Bantam, 1990.
- ———.Creating Health. Boston: Houghton-Mifflin, 1987
- Clifford, 1984 referred to in Recognition of Pain and Distress in

- Laboratory Animals, "Control of Pain" published by the Institute of Laboratory Animal Resources, 1992.
- Cousins, Norman. Anatomy of an Illness from a Patient's Perspective. New York: Norton, 1979.
- Depraz, Natalie, Francisco Varela, and Pierre Vermersch. On Becoming Aware: A Pragmatics of Experiencing. Vol. 43 in Advances in Consciousness Research. John Benjamins Publishing Company, 2000.
- Dossey, Larry. Healing Words: The Power of Prayer and the Practice of Medicine. New York: HarperCollins, 1993.
- ———. Reinventing Medicine. New York: HarperCollins, 1999.
- ———. Meaning and Medicine. New York: Bantam, 1992.
- Dudjom Rinpoche. Counsels from My Heart. Boston: Shambhala, 2001.
- Eliade, Mircea. Shamanism: Archaic Techniques of Ecstasy. 1966.
- Freemantle, Francesca. Luminous Emptiness. Boston: Shambhala, 2001.
- Frölich, Herbert. "Coherent Excitations in Active Biological Systems." In Felix Gutmann and Hendrik Keyzer. Modern Bioelectrochemistry. New York: Plenum, 1986.
- Gabor, Mate. *When the Body Says No.* London: Wiley, 2003.
- Gerber, Richard. Vibrational Medicine. Santa Fe, NM: Bear, 1988.
- Goldsmith, Joel, Parentheses in Eternity, 1962
- Goleman, Daniel, and G. E. Schwartz. "Meditation as an Intervention in Stress Reactivity." Journal of Consulting and Clinical Psychology 44, no. 3 (1976): 456–66.
- Goleman, Daniel. Emotional Intelligence. New York: Bantam, 1995.
- Goswami, Amit. The Self-Aware Universe. New York: Tarcher/Putnam, 1993.
- Govindan, Marshall. Babaji and the 18 Siddha Kriya Yoga Tradition. Montreal: Kriya Yoga Publications, 1991.
- Green, Elmer, and Alyce Green. *Beyond Biofeedback.* New York: Dell, 1977
- Greiner, Walter, and Aurel Sandulescu. "New Radioactivities." Scientific American (March 1990).
- Hampden-Turner, Charles. Maps of the Mind. New York: Macmillan, 1982.
- Holmes, Ernest, The Science of Mind, Los Angeles: Institute of Religious Science, 1997.
- Hopkins, Emma Curtis. Esoteric Philosophy. Portland, OR: WiseWoman Press, 2009

General References

- Hudson, David. "Alchemy: Portland Presentation." Video. 1998.
- Institute of Noetic Sciences website: www.noetic.org
- Isherwood, Christopher, and Swami Prabhavananda. How to Know God. Los Angeles: Vedanta, 1953.
- Jacobson, Edmund. Progressive Relaxation. Chicago: University of Chicago Press, 1938.
- James, William. The Varieties of Religious Experience. New York: Doubleday & Co., 1978.
- Jampolsky, Gerald. Teach Only Love. Hillsboro, OR: Beyond Words, 1992.
- Johnson, Willard. Riding the Ox Home: A History of Meditation from Shamanism to Science, Boston: Beacon Press, 2008.
- Jung, Carl G. Memories, Dreams, Reflections: Life After Death. New York: Random House, 1961.
- Kabat-Zinn, Jon. Full Catastrophe Living. New York: Bantam-Doubleday, 1990.
- Kaptchuk, Ted J. The Web That Has No Weaver. New York: Congdon & Weed, 1983.
- Kennedy Winner, Anne. The Basic Ideas of Occult Wisdom, Theosophical Press, 1970.
- Kirsch, Irving. The Emperor's New Drugs, Harvard U. Press, & google ebooks, 2012
- Khalsa, Dharma S. Meditation as Medicine. New York: Simon & Schuster, 2001.
- Lawlis, G. Frank. Transpersonal Medicine. Boston: Shambhala, 1996.
- Lipton, Bruce. The Biology of Belief. Santa Rosa, CA: Elite Press, 2005.
- Lo, Pei-Chen, Ming-Liang Huang, and Kang-Ming Chang. "EEG Alpha Blocking Correlated with Perception of Inner Light During Zen Meditation." American Journal of Chinese Medicine 31, no. 4 (2003): 629–42.
- Magarey, C. "Anxiety, Fear, and Meditation." Medical Journal of Australia 1, no. 7 (1981): 375.
- Markley, Oliver W., and Willis Harman. Changing Images of Man. Menlo Park, CA: Stanford Research Institute, 1975; also New York: Pergamon, 1984.
- Masters, Robert, and Jean Houston. Mind Games. New York: Delta, 1972.
- McTaggart, Lynn. The Field, the quest for the secret force of the universe. New York: HarperCollins, 2009.
- Mead, G. R. S. The Doctrine of the Subtle Body in Western Tradition. Wheaton, IL: Quest, 1919, 1967.
- Medigrace website: www.medigrace.org

- Miller, Iona, and Richard Miller. "Biophysics/Mindbody." nexusmagazine. com, 2004.
- Miller, Ruth L. 150 Years of Healing. Portland, OR: Abib, 1999.
- Mindell, Arnold, Working With the Dreaming Body. London, England. Penguin-Arkana//Lao Tse Press, 2000.
- Murphy, Michael. The Future of the Body. Los Angeles: Tarcher, 1992.
- _____, and Steven Donovan. The Physical and Psychological Effects of Meditation. Sausalito, CA: IONS, 1999.
- Myss, Caroline. The Anatomy of the Spirit. New York: Harmony Books, 1994.
- Myss, Caroline.Why People Don't Heal, and How They Can. New York: Harmony Books, 1997.
- Ornish, Dean, website: www.ornish.com.
- _____. Program for Reversing Heart Disease. New York: Random House, 1990.
- Ornstein, Robert. Psychology of Consciousness. New York: Viking, 1972.
- Oschman, James. Energy Medicine: The Scientific Basis. London: Churchill, 2000.
- Ouspensky, P. D. In Search of the Miraculous. New York: Harcourt, 1949.
- Pearce, Joseph Chilton, & Thom Hartmann. The Crack in the Cosmic Egg. New York: Julian Press, 1971.
- Pelletier, Kenneth. Mind as Healer/Mind as Slayer. New York: Dell, 1975.
- Pert, Candace. *Molecules of Emotion*. New York: Touchstone, 1997.Physical Review Letters 62, no. 10 (March 6, 1989).
- Popp, Fritz-Albert. "Physical Aspects of Biophotons." Experientia 44 (1988): 576–85.
- Prigogine, Ilya, and Stern. Order Out of Chaos. Toronto: Bantam, 1984.
- Puthoff, Harold E. "Everything for Nothing." New Scientist (July 28, 1990).
- Rama, Swami, Rudolph Ballentine, and Alan Hymes. Science of Breath. Honesdale, PA: Himalayan International Institute, 1979.
- Ramacharaka, The Hindu-Yogi Science Of Breath, project Gutenberg
- Reiter, Russel, and Jo Robinson. Melatonin: Your Body's Natural Wonder Drug. New York: Bantam, 1995.
- Remen, Rachel Naomi. Kitchen Table Wisdom, Riverhead Books, 2006.
- Schlitz, Marilyn, et al. Consciousness and Healing. St. Louis, MO: Elsevier, 2005.

General References

- Sheldrake, Rupert. A New Science of Life. Los Angeles: Tarcher, 1981.
- _____, Terence McKenna, and Ralph Abraham. The Evolutionary Mind. Santa Cruz, CA: Trialogue Press, 1998.
- Shinn, Florence Scovel. The Game of Life and How to Play It, (various publishers) or Ruth Miller's The NEW Gave of Life and How to Play It, New York: Simon & Schuster, 2012.
- Shrock, Dean, Why Love Heals: Mind-Body-Spirit Medicine. Eagle Point, OR: Heartfelt Intent Publications, 2009.
- Sogyal Rinpoche. The Tibetan Book of Living and Dying. New York: HarperCollins, 1994.
- Suzuki, D. T. An Introduction to Zen Buddhism. New York: Harper & Row, 1949.
- _____. Zen Buddhism. New York: Doubleday, 1956.
- Swanson, Claude. Life Force; The Scientific Basis. Poseida Press, 2009.
- Targ, Russell, and Jane Katra. Miracles of Mind. Novato, CA: New World Library, 1999.
- Tart, Charles. Altered States of Consciousness. New York: Wiley, 1969.
- _____. States of Consciousness. New York: Dutton, 1975.
- Thinley Norbu. The Small Golden Key. New York: Jewel, 1985.
- Thondup, Tulku. The Practice of Dzogchen: Writings of Longchen Rabjam. Ithaca, NY: Snow Lion, 1989.
- Transcendental Meditation website: www.tm.org.
- Trungpa, Chogyam. Glimpses of Abidharma. Boston: Shambhala, 1978.
- Weintraub, Michael I. "Qigong and Neurologic Illness." published in Alternative and Complementary Treatments in Neurologic Illness, New York: Elsevier, 2001.
- Wilcock, David, The Source Field Investigations, New York: Dutton/Penguin, 2011.
- Winner, Anne Kennedy. The Basic Ideas of Occult Wisdom. Wheaton, IL: Quest, 1970.
- Wirth, D. 1990. "The Effect of Non-Contact Therapeutic Touch on the Healing of Full Thickness Dermal Wounds." Subtle Energies 1 (1990).
- Yogananda, Paramahansa. Autobiography of a Yogi, Self-Realization Fellowship, Los Angeles, 1950; 2011
- Zohar, Danah. The Quantum Self: Human Nature and Consciousness Defined by the New Physics. New York: William Morrow, 1990.

Index

Achterberg, Jeanne.... 21, 138, 300, 303, 309
acupuncture ... 2, 26, 106, 109, 124, 141, 142
AIDS . 8, 25, 35, 43, 45, 54, 57, 66, 146, 147, 221, 222, 326
alaya 89, 90, 291
American Medical Association 1, 2, 299, 309
anxiety ... 1, 19, 24, 46, 47, 53, 54, 55, 57-59, 62, 63-65, 68-73, 86, 146, 182, 191, 258, 326
ASC, altered state of consciousness 80
astral body................. 123, 124
attention13, 19, 31, 35, 39, 46, 47, 48, 55, 57, 61, 64, 65, 67, 81, 88, 91, 93, 136, 147, 151, 153, 159, 163, 166, 168, 171, 182, 199, 201, 205, 209, 222, 234, 237, 243, 264, 271, 275
audio-guides 149, 235
awareness...ii, 3, 7, 16, 17, 20, 21, 27, 28, 37, 39, 40, 46-49, 53, 55, 57, 61, 63, 65, 67, 72, 79-81, 83, 88-92, 101, 106, 111, 118, 121, 124-128, 133, 139, 141, 145, 148, 149, 151, 153, 159, 164, 166, 169, 174, 176-179, 181-185, 189-197, 199, 206, 215, 219, 224, 229, 235-237, 240-243, 250, 259, 261, 271, 272, 275, 278-280, 289-291, 294, 298
Ayurveda 38, 39, 40
belief 10, 12, 102, 299, 304, 309, 311
Benson, Herbert... 1, 4, 51, 53, 56, 58, 65, 68, 70, 139, 158, 182, 258, 273, 299, 302, 303, 306, 307, 309
bindu 106, 125, 291, 294
biofeedback (BF) 18-20, 72, 300, 310
biophysics 4, 8
Borysenko, Joan...... 51, 56, 57, 302, 309
breathing37, 46-48, 54, 55, 61, 67, 99-101, 111, 143, 145, 146, 147, 170-172, 181-192, 196, 201, 205, 216, 222, 223, 225, 238, 255, 258, 274, 277, 290, 292-295, 323
British Society for Psychical Research........................ 122
Buddha-nature. 127, 128, 279, 289, 294
Buddhism ...iii, 40, 41, 42, 44, 46, 101, 110, 251, 272, 277, 290, 294, 297, 301, 313, 323
Buddhist.. 7, 29, 40-46, 53, 54, 86-90, 97, 105, 110, 125-128, 130, 143, 181, 221, 223, 249, 265, 277, 293, 297, 301, 302, 323
Bum Chung 110, 290
CAM, Complementary and Alternative Medicine... 2, 4, 19, 95, 274, 290
cancer care 4, 9, 21, 22, 25, 34, 36, 39, 54, 55, 57, 65, 66, 68, 70-72, 146, 182, 221, 222, 326

Index

cardiovascular care.. 4, 65, 66, 68, 69
Castaneda, Carlos................ 7
causal body........ 123, 124, 127
cell walls as semiconductors 102
cells as liquid crystals 104, 111
chakras 65, 105, 106, 107, 111, 294
chi 66, 95, 99-101, 109, 110, 111, 133, 142, 181, 183, 277, 278, 290, 292
childbirth 4, 43, 146, 147, 182, 221, 258, 275, 323, 326
Chopra, Deepak .. 8, 9, 12, 25, 38, 39, 67, 74, 111, 299, 301, 303, 309
Christian Science 32, 122, 259
Christianity.. 29, 93, 120, 121, 301
Collective Consciousness. 116, 118
continuum of consciousness 82, 93, 133, 136
Cousins, Norman . 11, 13, 299, 306, 310
cybernetics............. 4, 8, 23, 84
depression... 57, 58, 62, 69, 70, 72, 146
Detsen, King Trisong.......... 41
Dharmakaya 90, 126-128, 133, 141, 265, 278, 287, 290-294
DHEA 64, 66
diabetes care 73
discrete states of consciousness.................. 82
disease 3, 18, 21, 39, 43, 44, 54, 55, 59-61, 65-71, 122, 130, 146-148, 157-159, 185, 207, 224, 230, 236, 249, 289, 299, 300
dissipative structures 97, 112, 131
Dossey, Larry 3, 5, 12, 95, 136, 221, 303, 306, 307, 310
Dreamtime........................ 272
drugs 1, 12, 62, 63, 80, 82, 151, 153, 249, 274
Dudjom *Rinpoche* 45, 297, 299, 302, 310, 323
Elmer and Alyce Green...... 18
Emoto, Masaru 103, 304
endorphins 63, 67
energy body . 65, 104-106, 125, 126, 134, 136, 142, 143, 145-147, 152, 153, 167, 179, 181-185, 196, 235, 271, 277, 279, 290, 293-295
energy medicine 142, 143, 151, 152, 185, 251, 290, 323
Era I . 3, 15, 95, 134, 143, 148, 236, 249, 251, 257
Era II 3, 4, 5, 95, 134, 143, 153, 275
Era III... 3, 4, 5, 134, 143, 150, 152, 154, 249, 275
etheric body............... 123, 124
Europe......... 8, 26, 42, 45, 292
fields . 4, 8, 17, 43, 80, 95, 108, 111-119, 129-133, 136, 141-143, 148, 152, 160, 166, 167, 175, 247, 264, 265, 267, 268, 271, 277, 290
Fremantle, Francesca.. 4, 106, 126-128, 297, 304, 305
Frölich, Herbert 108, 109, 310
Gampo, King Strongtsan.... 40
Gerber, Richard 105, 123-125, 304-306, 310
Goswami, Amit .. 14, 101, 111, 126, 267, 305, 310
Grossinger, Richard...... 2, 324
Gurdjieff, Georges 84, 85, 126, 304
Harvard Medical Center 4, 51, 53, 54, 157, 158
Hay, Louise 13, 34, 35
healing as part of being

Christian 30
healthcare alternatives 273
health-care industry 275
Hindu...i, 7, 29, 36, 37, 40, 45,
  46, 58, 65, 86, 87, 89, 105,
  125, 181, 265, 267, 270, 277,
  295, 301, 304, 312
Hinduism 36, 101, 301
ho'oponopono 139
Holling, C.S. 260
holograms 119
Hopkins, Emma Curtis. 33-36,
  137, 301, 310, 325
hormones 55, 64, 66
Houston, Jean .. 20, 22, 23, 85,
  199, 311
illness. 1, 11, 13, 33-35, 48, 86,
  124, 136, 137, 140, 144, 147,
  207, 226, 229, 255, 258, 259,
  261, 281, 289
imagery 11, 16, 20-23, 80, 129,
  135, 139, 142-144, 152, 183,
  199, 200, 207, 258
immune system. 12, 64-67, 71,
  184, 224
India 36, 38, 40, 42, 51, 54, 89,
  266
Institute of Heartmath 17
InteliHealth 18, 19
intention ... 2, 5, 15, 18, 21, 25,
  48, 103, 127, 138-143, 146,
  183, 209, 217, 225, 228, 229,
  269-271, 276, 281
IONS, Institute of Noetic
  Sciences 17, 24, 25, 312
Islam 45, 92, 120, 301
Jampolsky, Gerald... 149, 150,
  306, 311
Journey to Wild Divine 20
Judaism 31, 92, 120, 121
Jung, Carl... 83, 117, 118, 133,
  148, 237, 306, 311
Kabat-Zinn, Jon 53, 54, 55, 56,
  62, 144, 158, 302, 306, 311

Khalsa, Dharma Singh MD 99,
  107, 304, 311
Krieger, Delores 15
kriya yoga 38, 89, 100, 272
Lawlis, Frank... 4, 22, 23, 138,
  139, 144, 300, 306, 311
laying on of hands.. 14, 24, 29,
  141
Len, Hew 139
Lipton, Bruce 10, 13, 102, 299,
  304, 311
Living Systems Theory 96
Lo, Pei-Chen 99, 110, 304, 305,
  311
luminous awareness 128
lung 72, 100, 101, 109, 111,
  133, 277-279, 292
Maharishi Effect... iii, 60, 270,
  272
Maharishi Mahesh Yogi ... 45,
  58, 272
Maret, Karl 102, 103, 104, 113,
  119, 305
Maté, Gabor 13, 152, 207
Mayo Clinic 19
medicine, history of 11
meditation (See awareness,
  attention, breathing,
  mindfulness)
melatonin 64-66
mental body 123, 250, 252
mental healing 13
mindfulness... i, 46, 47, 48, 49,
  53, 54, 63, 145, 292, 298
MIT (Massachusetts Institute
  of Technology) 63, 64
molecules of emotion 9, 111
Morphic Resonance... 116-118,
  265
Murphy, Michael 4, 10, 11, 19,
  20, 62, 70, 71, 199, 264, 299-
  303, 306, 307, 312
Myss, Caroline 3, 104, 136, 258
National Institutes of Health 2,

Index

9, 25, 101, 274
near-death care 4, 43, 146, 249, 258
neuropeptides 9, 10
New Thought 7, 32, 34, 35, 121, 122, 150, 151, 259, 301, 325
Nirmanakaya... 126, 128, 290, 294
Ornish, Dean 60, 61, 145, 302, 303, 312
Oschman, James 113, 304, 305, 312
Padmasambhava.. 41, 43, 251, 290, 292, 297, 298, 301
Padre Pio 30
pain management .. 53, 54, 62, 63, 73, 146, 159
paradigm .... iii, 2, 3, 257, 273, 292
Patanjali ... 37, 38, 87, 88, 301, 309
Pelletier, Kenneth 67, 70, 302, 303, 307, 312
Pert, Candace 9, 299, 312
placebo 11, 25, 26
prana .. 36, 37, 61, 95, 99, 100, 101, 106, 109, 111, 125, 133, 142, 181, 277, 278
prayer 29, 30, 33, 56, 121, 139, 152, 153, 270, 271
Prigogine, Ilya 97-99, 101, 304, 312
Progressive Relaxation 48, 138, 144, 152, 157, 200, 258, 309, 311
psychoneuroimmunology 8
psychosomatic 12
Qi Gong, (also *chi gung*, *ki-gung*) 16, 25
quantum physics ... 4, 8, 9, 266
Quimby, Phineas P. 13, 32, 35, 137
receptors 10, 102
Reiki 15, 26, 141, 142, 153, 292

Relaxation Response ... 56, 57, 139, 309
Releasing the Past ii, 207, 271
resonant pattern 118, 129
rigpa 89, 90, 92, 133, 183, 261, 280, 283, 28-291, 304
Ron Roth 31
Sambhogakaya . 126-128, 132, 141, 290, 291, 293, 294
Schumann's Resonances . 115, 116
scientific medicine 1, 3, 25, 101, 134, 135, 150, 259
self-care .... vii, 4, 56, 129, 134, 135, 140-143, 151, 158, 159, 201, 221, 235, 238, 257, 258, 262, 273, 275, 276, 292
shamanic traditions 24, 27, 28, 109, 111, 151, 259
shaman 7, 27, 28, 114, 137, 259, 272, 299
Sheldrake, Rupert 116-118, 264, 265, 305, 313
Simonton, Carl 21, 199
Spiritualist churches 121, 122
states of consciousness 28, 59, 80-83, 85, 88, 93, 115, 136, 137
stillpoint 48
subtle body 106, 123, 125, 128, 293
suffering ... 22, 46, 47, 63, 140, 146-148, 160, 161, 195, 221-232, 271
Suzuki, D.T. 45, 313
Swanson, Claude . 4, 109, 141, 304, 313
Tart, Charles T. 63, 79-82, 84-86, 92, 93, 303, 304, 313
terma 43, 290
Therapeutic Touch. 15, 16, 26, 141, 300, 313
Tibet ... i, 40-44, 114, 146, 221, 251, 290, 294, 298, 301

Tibetan, 29, 40-45, 47, 53, 86, 89, 90, 100, 101, 106, 127, 181, 221, 250, 251, 277, 280, 289, 291, 295-299, 301, 302, 304, 307, 313, 323-325
Tong Len 146, 323
trance states 21, 28, 29
Transcendental Meditation, TM .45, 46, 58-60, 271, 302, 313
Transformative Compassionate Breathing 141, 146, 223, 229, 231, 271
transpersonal 3, 21, 23, 25, 83, 136, 138, 150, 153, 221, 223, 233, 236, 263-265
trikaya 126, 128, 133, 271, 279
Tsogyal, Yeshe ... 43, 294, 297, 298, 301
Tulku ... 43, 127, 297, 298, 313
UCLA University of California at Los Angeles 64
UMMC, University of Massachusetts Medical Center.53-55, 61-65, 68, 71, 158
Upanishads 7, 87, 125
Vajrayana Buddhism....iii, 41, 44, 45, 53, 101, 181, 251, 272, 277, 279, 280, 290, 291, 294, 297
Vase Breathing 110, 145, 146, 152, 153, 182-185, 189, 190, 193-196, 279, 290, 292, 294, 295
Vedas 36, 65, 87, 105
Vedic traditions 7, 36
Vipashyana 46, 47, 54, 67, 294, 323
visualization 21, 22, 24, 72, 85, 89, 93, 138, 183, 199, 200, 295, 323
waking consciousness .. 82, 85, 258
wellness rememberd 273
Yoga 36, 37, 38, 86, 87, 88, 295, 309, 310
Yogananda, Paramahansa 38, 88, 89, 100, 301, 313
yogis 36, 52, 53, 86, 87, 259
Zen 20, 45, 52, 53, 67, 110, 181, 291, 311, 313
Zohar, Danah ... 111, 266, 267, 285, 287, 304, 307, 313

Acknowledgements

Robert's Acknowledgements

First and foremost, this book would not exist if it wasn't for Dr. Ruth Miller. I had started work on this project in 2002 and had drafted half the book, but I was overwhelmed with commitments in my childbirth meditation work and I would never have finished this project. Actually something like an angel, Ruth liked my vision for the book and saw it as chance to advance her research in physical and spiritual sciences. She accepted my offer to work as partners in a book that was to disclose the great background of the use of meditation in healing, the current scope of its use in mind-body medicine, a new model of the human body appropriate for advances in mind-body and energy medicine, and a new model of health and healthcare. As we worked together to utilize the most important research, we evolved a language that was so much our own we still can't tell who wrote what. Our combined energies went beyond what either of us could have done alone, and after 10 years of exciting work we have finished a big offering, presented to help build a better world. Thank you forever Ruth.

A most important inspiration for me behind the creation of this book is H. H. Dudjom Rinpoche, former head of the Nyingma lineage of Tibetan Buddhism. His personal guidance and teachings on the nature of the mind and body are my greatest resource. His son and lineage heir, H. H. Shenphen Dawa Rinpoche, was my teacher and trainer for the vase breathing and some of the visualization methods presented in this book. The teachings, transmissions, and empowerments of Dudjom Rinpoche and Shenphen Rinpoche have remained a special source of grace to me in my work in the medical establishment. I'll be forever grateful.

The meditation master Chogyam Trungpa Rinpoche, my first lama, with whom I worked from 1970 to 1980, inspired me to practice Vipashyana meditation and Tong Len sincerely for 10 years, and was a great model for how to teach Buddhist psychological methods in the West.

We wish to thank Gerald Lehrburger, MD, chairman of the Board of Medigrace and president of Health Research Institute for his important support in helping Medigrace evolve.

When Ruth and I were finishing this document for publication, the book received another grace. Anna Humphreys stepped up to the computer and saved us from doing hours of mechanical work needed to finish the book. Anna got excited and told me it was a masterpiece. Thank you, Anna!

Ruth's Acknowledgements

Throughout my career, I've been deeply appreciative of the opportunity to integrate the wisdom of the ancients with the discoveries of the present, and in this particular work, that's been even more the case. From the day that Robert heard me lecture on the new sciences and emerging understandings about healing, then asked me to consider working with him on this book, this has been a remarkable learning process. Becoming familiar with the Tibetan methods and model, and with the many years of meditation research that have gone on in this country and their results, then integrating those into the emerging model of healing, has been an delightful deepening of my understanding. Thank you Robert for making it possible.

Thanks also go to Richard Grossinger for encouraging and publishing the first edition of this work, and to the members of The Portal Center and of Medigrace for making this second edition, with its new information and format, possible.

About the Authors

Robert Bruce Newman is Executive Director of Medigrace. He studied, practiced, and was trained to teach under the guidance of Tibetan meditation teachers and doctors for more than 20 years, from 1970 onwards. He was trained in a new and more complete model of the human body than Western medicine has been based on. From 1995 to the present he has directed more than 100 hospital trainings in the medical uses of meditation. He has presented at the University of Michigan Medical School and four times at the world congress of the Association of Prenatal and Perinatal Psychology and Health (APPPAH). His books include: *Calm Birth; New Method for Conscious Childbirth* (2005); *Calm Healing; Methods for a New Era of Medicine* (2006) with Ruth L. Miller; and *Transforming Childbirth; the Calm Birth Method* (2012).

Ruth L. Miller is currently Research Director at The Portal Center for the Unification of Psyche, Science, and Spirit, followng overlapping 20-year careers as a futurist/college professor and a New Thought minister. Her degrees in anthropology, environmental studies, cybernetic systems, and systems science have focused on the nature and role of human consciousness in our culture. Her classes integrate modern science with ancient wisdom for a clearer understanding and better life. Most of her books bring the teachings of early New Thought leaders and healers into modern language with modern examples. Some recent titles include: *Unveiling Your Hidden Power, Emma Curtis Hopkins' Metaphysics for the 21st Century; Natural Abundance, Ralph Waldo Emerson's Guide for Prosperity;* and *As We Think So We Are, James Allen's guide for transforming our lives.*

About Medigrace

Medigrace was founded in New York City in 1991 by Robert Bruce Newman, Dr. Ted Wolff of New York University Medical Center Research, and Drs. Craig Spaniol and John Sutton of NASA. The intent was to research and develop programs advancing the use of meditation in medicine and in childbirth. The program moved to Ashland, Oregon, in 1995 and began to work with several Southern Oregon Hospitals, including Rogue Valley Medical Center (Medford), and Providence Medford Medical Center. The original programs were of two kinds: meditation for stress management for health care providers, for their own health, and programs using meditation for pain and anxiety management, cancer care, and HIV-AIDS care. In 1998-99 Medigrace worked with the California health care system, with the support of Sutter Health. By 2000 the response to Calm Birth, the Medigrace childbirth meditation program, was such that all resources and focus went into that practice for the next decade. In 2009 Christine Novak, RN, HNC, director of the Calm Birth program, was awarded the March of Dimes Better-for-Baby nursing award for bringing the Calm Birth program into the New Jersey hospital system. To date hundreds of teachers have been trained in the Calm Birth method, and through it more than 12,000 children have been born, representing a higher standard of maternal ad infant health.

About Calm Birth

For information about the Calm Birth program, products and services, please visit the Calm Birth web site: www.calmbirth.org

www.medigrace.org
223 Fifth St. ste B Ashland, Oregon 97520 USA

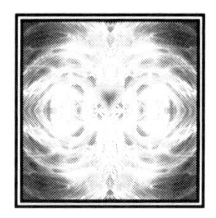

A
MEDIGRACE
Book

published by Portal Center Press
www.portalcenterpress.com

MedigraceBooks was established with the 2012 publication of this book, *Empowered Care; Mind-Body Medicine Methods*, and a new manual for Childbirth based on the Calm Birth Method. Medigrace Books will continue to publish titles that demonstrate a better way for children to be born and a better way to practice health care.